Contraceptiv|

ST. MICHAEL'S PARTNERSHIP
ST. MICHAEL'S SURGERY
WALWYN CLOSE
TWERTON
BATH BA2 1ER
TEL: 01225 428277

PSYCHOSEXUAL MEDICINE SERIES
Edited by Ruth L. Skrine MB, ChB, MRCGP

Psychosexual Medicine is a discipline which uses a combined body and mind approach to problems related to sexuality, and which stresses the importance of the doctor–patient relationship. The method derives from psychoanalysis but is distinct in that the practitioner listens to unconscious material over a focused, narrow field. The work of many doctors and nurses, and of some physiotherapists, provides opportunities for physical examination and treatment of the genital area which are unavailable to non-medical sexual therapists. Both physical and psychological problems and the interaction between them can be explored at the time of physical examination.

This series forms part of the developing body of knowledge held by members of the Institute of Psychosexual Medicine, formed in London in 1974. The books are for doctors and their colleagues who are interested in a psychosomatic approach to sexual problems particularly those working in general practice and gynaecology, as well as psychological and genito-urinary medicine.

Contraceptive Care
Meeting individual needs

Edited by

HEATHER MONTFORD

MB, BS, DRCOG, Mem. Inst. Psychosexual Medicine
Senior Clinical Medical Officer
Family Planning and Psychosexual Medicine
Margaret Pyke Centre
London

and

RUTH SKRINE

MB, ChB, MRCGP, Mem. Inst. Psychosexual Medicine
Senior Clinical Medical Officer
Family Planning and Psychosexual Medicine
Bath and Bristol

CHAPMAN & HALL
London · Glasgow · New York · Tokyo · Melbourne · Madras

Published by Chapman & Hall, 2–6 Boundary Row, London SE1 8HN

Chapman & Hall, 2–6 Boundary Row, London SE1 8HN, UK

Blackie Academic & Professional, Wester Cleddens Road, Bishopbriggs, Glasgow G64 2NZ, UK

Chapman & Hall Inc., 29 West 35th Street, New York NY10001, USA

Chapman & Hall Japan, Thomson Publishing Japan, Hirakawacho Nemoto Building, 6F, 1-7-11 Hirakawa-cho, Chiyoda-ku, Tokyo 102, Japan

Chapman & Hall Australia, Thomas Nelson Australia, 102 Dodds Street, South Melbourne, Victoria 3205, Australia

Chapman & Hall India, R. Seshadri, 32 Second Main Road, CIT East, Madras 600 035, India

Distributed in the USA and Canada by Singular Publishing Group Inc., 4284 41st Street, San Diego, California 92105

First edition 1993

© 1993 Chapman & Hall

Typeset by Mews Photosetting, Beckenham, Kent
Printed in Great Britain by Page Bros (Norwich) Ltd.

ISBN 0 412 47050 0   1 56593 213 7 (USA)

A catalogue record for this book is available from the British Library

Library of Congress Cataloging-in-Publication data available

∞ Printed on permanent acid-free text paper, manufactured in accordance with the proposed ANSI/NISO Z 39.48-199X and ANSI Z 39.48-1984

Contents

Contents

Contributors

Pauline Allen MB BS MRCS LRCP DRCOG, Mem. Inst. Psychosexual Medicine, manager family planning services, Gloucester

Alessandra Bispham MB ChB MRCPsych, Mem. Inst. Psychosexual Medicine, senior clinical medical officer family planning and psychosexual medicine, London

Elphis Christopher MB BS DRCOG DCH, Mem. Inst. Psychosexual Medicine, senior clincal medical officer family planning and psychosexual medicine, London

Elaine Cooper MB ChB MRCS LRCP, Ass. Inst. Psychosexual Medicine, director of family planning services, Southampton

Bozena Davies MB ChB, Mem. Inst. Psychosexual Medicine, sessional doctor, Brook Advisory Centre, Birmingham

Heather Montford MB BS DRCOG, Mem. Inst. Psychosexual Medicine, senior clinical medical officer family planning and psychosexual medicine, Margaret Pyke Centre, London

Ann Morgan MB BS DRCOG DCH, Mem. Inst. Psychosexual Medicine, senior clinical medical officer family planning and psychosexual medicine, Cheltenham

Roseanna Pollen MB BS MRCGP, Mem. Inst. Psychosexual Medicine, general practitioner, London

Merryl Roberts MB ChB, Mem. Inst. Psychosexual Medicine, senior clinical medical officer family planning and psychosexual medicine, Canterbury

Sam Rowlands MRCGP DCH DRCOG, general practitioner, Biggleswade, Bedfordshire

Ruth Skrine MB ChB MRCGP, Mem. Inst. Psychosexual Medicine, senior clinical medical officer family planning and psychosexual medicine, Bath and Bristol

Andrew Stainer-Smith MA MRCP MRCGP, Mem. Inst. Psychosexual Medicine, general practitioner, Okehampton, Devon

Beryl Tully MB ChB, Mem. Inst. Psychosexual Medicine, senior clinical medical officer family planning and psychosexual medicine, Bristol

Gill Wakley MB ChB, Mem. Inst. Psychosexual Medicine, general practitioner, Kidsgrove, North Staffordshire

Foreword

Professor Robert Snowden
Professor of Family Studies, University of Exeter

It is not long since the medical profession was expelling those of its members who openly suggested that doctors should assist in providing a safe and effective contraceptive service for patients. But Dr Albert Arbuthnot, who was barred from practising medicine in 1885 for stating such a belief, would probably be surprised at the speed and degree of change that has occurred since his historic stand. Now it is unthinkable to consider a family planning service without the involvement of doctors. Why is this and what does it presage for the future activities of doctors and other health care professionals working in this specialty?

Doctors did not become involved in contraceptive provision because of a direct interest in the prevention of births, but rather as an indirect attempt to reduce the deleterious consequences of excess births on the health of those directly and indirectly involved. The earliest medical records I have seen are of women attending the family planning clinics in a rural area (Devon) at a time of considerable rural poverty in the early 1930s. It came as something of a shock to learn that prolapse of the womb was commonplace, that tuberculosis among the women and their families was endemic, and that women in their early 20s had often already experienced six or more confinements (usually accompanied by a high infant mortality rate). It is therefore not surprising that medical advisers faced with these problems have made considerable efforts over the years to promote freely available and efficient contraceptive care as a humanitarian objective.

In the 1930s various barrier methods were available. The development of spermicides had, by then, also made a hesitant beginning, but only a few doctors were aware of the Grafenberg Ring, the first generally available intrauterine device (IUCD). For family planning to be effective at that time much depended on the volition and perseverance of the user. The relationship between the patient, doctor and the technology developed from the desire to provide the necessary personal support for those in obvious need. Because the contraceptive technology was in a relatively primitive stage of development, emphasis was placed on encouraging those who wished to plan their families, and such encouragement required some understanding of the emotional and sexual lives of the users. Family planning pioneers were usually perceived as 'enthusiasts' who saw their work in humanitarian terms and who were often involved in other activities concerned with the emancipation of women. In other words, the satisfaction of the needs and the understanding of the feelings of the individual user were the desired end results, with the available technology being seen as a means to that end.

However, a change took place during the 1950s and 1960s when a surge in contraceptive technological development coincided with a perceived need to control the rapid rate of population growth. The call for global population control and the institution of large-scale family planning programmes – usually aimed at the populations of developing countries – gave added impetus to this development. This emphasis on a technological 'fix' tended to obscure the equally important need to study the factors affecting the *acceptability* of the technology being developed.

With the arrival of this contraceptive technology, new techniques in the collection and interpretation of data relating to its use were introduced, together with a distinctive and specialized language. New words were used to explain the difference in effectiveness of the same type of contraceptive used by different groups of people. Those of us familiar with the family planning scene during this period soon came across such words as 'theoretical effectiveness' and 'use-effectiveness'. Theoretical effectiveness, we were told, described the use of a product exactly according to instructions and is therefore the 'true' rate, whereas use-effectiveness describes the rate of unwanted pregnancies in terms of the experience of couples using the product during the emotional and physical somersaults of their love-life. Such a distinction is important when the primary aim is the promotion of a product which can be presented as highly effective 'if only it were used properly'. This over-riding concern with the promotion of the product inevitably reduces emphasis on the needs of the contraceptive user. If a pregnancy results it is not the technology that is at fault but the poor use being made of it by its users! The search for a technical answer to a social 'problem' was very pronounced during these decades, at a time when there appeared to be a general consensus that the answer to the planet's population problem lay in the inventive ability of the biomedical scientist.

But the pendulum was beginning to swing back. There was a growing awareness that success in terms of reducing the birth rate was not as great as might be expected from the new technology, and that while the various methods became more available, their general acceptance often remained elusive. It is true that individuals (and some international organizations such as the International Planned Parenthood Federation and the Population Council) had been advocating the need to understand the personal and social factors influencing contraceptive use. However, it was not until the setting up of the Acceptabilty Task Force by the World Health Organisation in the early 1970s (to be renamed the Psychosocial Task Force about 10 years later), that the relevance of psychology and sociology to the study of contraceptive use and provision was formally recognized by the medical profession.

The most obvious and perhaps important characteristic of contraceptive behaviour is that it is generally disliked, in marked contrast to the sexual behaviour which prompts its need. Herein lies the perpetual conflict between those who provide and those who use contraceptives. Those who choose to use contraceptives do not do so in any sense of favourable anticipation. There is nothing positive about the choice. Indeed, while choice is present it is based on a negative discrimination. Contraceptives are used because not using them is perceived to have a higher cost than the inconvenience and dislike of using them. In this sense putting on a condom or inserting a cap; having an IUD fitted; using spermicides; taking systemic drugs or resorting to surgery are not activities that anyone would seek positively.

This negative approach to the subject matter has disadvantages for those of us who have spent our professional lives attempting to improve family planning provision. We can envy our colleagues who services are valued more positively. Because there is nothing intrinsically pleasant about contraception, we can never hope to provide a completely acceptable service. The most we can do is to provide a service which reduces the level of unacceptabilty to the minimum. This means that success will always be relative and never absolute.

We have, then, a service which most users would prefer to avoid and which requires behaviour of a negative kind. An additional complication is that a factor which may be unacceptable to one person poses no problem to another. Much will depend on factors such as age, past reproductive and contraceptive experience and reproductive intentions. There is a further aspect which is infrequently discussed, which tends to embarrass, which requires a level of personal awareness many do not possess, and which is replete with social and personal taboos of a significant kind. I refer to the fact that contraceptive behaviour is intimately associated with sexual behaviour. The possession of knowledge about the blood pressure or previous menstrual patterns among Pill or IUCD users is clearly important, but in terms of the successful use of these methods and of the medical care of the whole woman, other factors are vital. These include such things as the number of sexual partners, the frequency of intercourse, the users' ideas about the methods, and most importantly their perception of their own needs. While providers of family planning services tend to concentrate on aspects of behaviour likely to enhance or detract from the effective use of specific contraceptive methods, users tend to view such technology in terms of needs associated with their sexual lives. Contraceptive technology is not normally viewed by users in an objective, clinical manner but within the context of an erotic and emotional experience.

The provision of an acceptable (and therefore effective) family planning service requires a wide range of skills which the health care professional is in the best position to provide. Success does not lie in technology alone but its use, combined with the sensitive handling of what for most people is a deeply personal, private and important matter, can result in a sense of satisfaction for the service user, and professional fulfilment for the provider. This book will do much to help health care professionals to understand and meet the complex and varied needs of women and men seeking advice about contraceptive care, and to play their part in the creation of healthy and planned families. Dr Arbuthnot would probably have been among the first to give it his endorsement.

About the Institute of Psychosexual Medicine

Information about seminar training for doctors can be obtained from:

The Institute of Psychosexual Medicine
11 Chandos Street
Cavendish Square
London W1M 9DE (tel. 071-580 0631)

Basic training normally lasts for two years and consists of fortnightly meetings in term-time. Each meeting lasts for two hours.

Doctors wishing to make this subject a specialty and become full members of the Institute will usually require at least two or three more years of seminar training before they are ready to appear before the examination panel.

Training in psychosexual nursing is in a state of evolution, and interested nurses should enquire through the English National Board for Nursing, Midwifery and Health Visiting, Victory House, 170 Tottenham Road, London W1P OHA (tel. 071-388 3131).

1

Unconscious factors in contraceptive care: understanding ambivalence and poor motivation

Elphis Christopher

SUMMARY

- Historical and political attitudes to fertility
- Contraceptive signs of conflict
- Pressures on the doctor
- The importance of mothers
- The feeling behind the symptom
- Conflict in the relationship
- Caring for the poorly motivated

The giving of contraceptive advice appears on the surface to be a straightforward and uncomplicated matter, consisting of two adults talking to each other. One is the patient, usually a woman coming for advice and guidance on which method to use, the other the doctor providing expert knowledge on benefits and risks.

However, contraceptive decisions involve all the facets of a person's life, not only as individuals in their personal relationships, but also within the wider context of their culture, religion and society. In current western society where sex is presented as a spontaneous, hot-blooded activity, thinking consciously about using contraception may be seen as cold, dampening the fires of passion. Sexually explicit scenes on the television, for example, rarely if ever mention the possibility of pregnancy or the use of contraception. The fact that many contraceptive consultations are straightforward can deceive the unwary doctor into thinking that they will all be simple. Where the consultation is not straightforward, it may be all too easy for the busy doctor to get caught up in the patient's internal conflicts. If this happens he may become irritated and impatient, reacting to the patient's behaviour, which on the surface appears unreasonable and inexplicable, rather than trying to understand what is behind it. The temptation will then be to suggest a change of contraceptive pill or a change of method, in the hope (usually forlorn) that the problem will be solved. In these situations the woman will either not return, or may return later with an unintended and possibly unwanted pregnancy.

The purpose of this chapter is to alert the doctor to the way unconscious conflicts, ambivalence and covert problems can present under the guise of a problem with contraception. It may well be inevitable, and indeed necessary, for the doctor to be caught up to some extent in the patient's conflict in order for it to be understood. Provided he or she can then step back and think about what is going on and suggest an interpretation for the patient, it may be possible for the conflict to be resolved.

HISTORICAL AND POLITICAL ATTITUDES TO FERTILITY

The decision to have a child must be the most fateful a person ever makes, involving as it does the creation of a new human being. Until comparatively recently in human history (the last 200 years), greater concern has been focused on fertility and the ability to have children to ensure the continuity of the human race, rather than the prevention of pregnancy. It is easy to lose sight of this historical legacy in the face of the problems to do with overpopulation. The barren woman unable to have children has always had a negative image. Thus the emphasis was on the ability to conceive. Fertility rites, spring festivals and the ancient fertility goddesses all bear witness to that (Neumann, 1955). All religions are pronatalist and anti-abortion, except in special circumstances. Couples were, and in some cases still are, urged 'to be fruitful and multiply', and 'to replenish the earth' as stated in the *Book of Genesis*. The purpose of sex was procreation and the gift of life was regarded as God-given. Riches were measured in the number of chlidren a couple had, especially sons.

National governments too are involved in individual decisions about fertility. Although there are 75 countries in which the birth rate is considered to be too high, there are still 21 where there are national policies aimed at increasing the number of births (United Nations, 1990).

However, deeply held cultural and religious traditions are often more powerful than political pressures, and they continue to influence individuals in much of the developing world and in certain ethnic groups from Asia and Africa in Britain. For example, there is a West Indian belief that a woman has a certain number of children inside her which she has to have and that nature should not be interfered with. We seek our immortality through our descendants, our children and our grandchildren. To thwart the possibility of conception can produce, at a deep psychic level, guilt about being anti-life and opposed to God. The words 'contraception' and 'birth control' sound hard and alienating, going against nature. Family planning, though less applicable to young people seeking advice on preventing pregnancy, has a softer ring to it. Although nowadays most people, certainly in the western world, do not want many children, and the benefits of contraception are self-evident, nevertheless there is a hidden psychic cost that is often denied but that can surface from time to time.

Thus to use contraception requires at some level a grieving for all the possible loved babies that could be born. We are all too aware of the terrible irony of couples assiduously and conscientiously using contraception for years, only to discover that one or other or both of them are infertile. An awareness of these often unspoken feelings may explain some of the enormous fear of the reliable methods of contraception that can underlie some contraceptive difficulties. Such methods are too powerful and will damage fertility. There is a fear of retribution, the woman will be unable to have children, and hence some will play contraceptive roulette in order to 'placate the gods'.

The reality, of course, has been that human beings from earliest historical times have tried to control their fertility when it was inconvenient to have a child. The sin of Onan in the *Old Testament* exemplifies this. Onan should under Hebraic law have impregnated his dead brother's wife. Instead he 'cast his seed upon the ground' angering God. This story has been used as evidence that all forms of non-reproductive sex and the use of contraception are against God's will. The ancient Egyptians used a vaginal pessary made of crocodile dung to prevent conception, and instruments to procure abortion were used in Roman times. Hippocrates, the father of medicine, advocated violent exercises. Thus powerful opposing forces are present in our psyches, both the urge to reproduce but also the urge to abort. All this may seem a far cry from the ordinary contraceptive consultation but every now and then these forces will be evident.

> Mrs A. did not believe in contraception, and although she said it was not because of her religion she said, 'It's just that you should have what God sends along and not interfere.' She was in her late 20s and had nine children from 12 pregnancies. After each pregnancy the use of contraception was suggested by the midwife, health visitor or doctor. Each time the answer was the same, and given in such a way that the professionals felt almost like child killers for even mentioning contraception. Eventually Mrs A. reached breaking point with her tenth child and a difficult delivery. Tired and worn out, she attended the doctor's surgery frequently for various ailments, both her own and those of her children. Finally, she managed to bring herself to ask for a sterilization. Fortunately, the doctor refrained form saying 'I told you so' and managed to expedite the operation in an understanding and friendly way.

This patient illustrates a well-known situation where the actual experience of childbirth and child rearing can change attitudes towards contraception. For Mrs A. there were further factors in her urge to have all the children she could have. She was the unwanted illegitimate child of a holiday romance and in her childhood she had been pushed around from pillar to post with no one to call her own. Her children were her bastion against the world, her own tribe as it were. Her sense that it was morally right to have what God sent fitted her unconscious inner need for a large family.

Religious views can also be used by a patient to explain to herself deep, unexpressed fears of the reliable contraceptive methods, as well as her ambivalent feelings about another baby that she may not fully recognize.

> Mrs B. was 23 years old, a strict Jehovah's Witness with three children under the age of three years. After a discussion about methods, she was adamant that she wanted no foreign chemicals in her body, and that she wished to rely on natural family planning, even although she insisted that she did not want another child for five years. She seemed unable to hear what the doctor said about the benefits and effectiveness of the oral contraceptive pill. The doctor, though tempted, felt that discretion was the better part of valour and did not persist in advocating a more reliable method. Instead she taught the woman how to predict ovulation using both the thermosymptal and mucus method. A year passed then Mrs B. became unintentionally pregnant. She could not contemplate an abortion. She had the child, a boy, which was what she wanted. After this pregnancy she decided to take no more chances. She opted for the contraceptive pill, which she has taken for six years without problems.

The occurrence of an unplanned pregnancy and the birth of another baby had produced a change in the way she perceived the various factors in her life. Her need for reliable contraception, and perhaps also the resolution of her ambivalence about wanting a boy, was strong enough to override her fear of chemicals and her religious influences.

CONTRACEPTIVE SIGNS OF CONFLICT

Contraceptive decisions are complicated, involving as they do the questions of whether to have children, the timing of such children and how many are wanted, as well as the choice of which contraceptive method and who should use it. Conflicts may manifest themselves in a variety of different ways. There can be a complaint or dissatisfaction with all methods. While such discontent may be legitimate in the sense that there is no perfect method, nevertheless most people do manage to make a choice. It may be necessary to confront the patient directly with a remark such as, 'It seems that no method is any good, and it is true we do not have the ideal method, but I was wondering if anything else was troubling you.' Such a remark can give the woman the necessary space to talk rather than forcing a choice upon her. She may have allowed herself to get frightened by the horror stories about the methods, exaggerating the dangers. She may feel she needs protecting against the risks of life itself and may wish she did not have to be grown up and take responsibility for her own actions. She may resent her partner's irresponsible attitude.

Complaints about a chosen method that had previously been satisfactory should not be taken at face value. Once medical reasons for the problem have been excluded the doctor must try to understand what other conflicts may be present. Similarly erratic use of a method, especially in a patient who has always been a regular user, should occasion concern and further exploration, in order to ascertain what is really going on in the patient's life. Older women, for instance, can begin to realize that the biological time clock is ticking away, and that they may have left the decision to have a baby too late. Sometimes they only want to know that they can get pregnant, and once they have done so they may request termination. A change from a reliable to a less reliable method may also reflect a covert wish to get pregnant even although that is denied consciously.

There may be a discrepancy between the strength of the patient's demand for contraception and her reliability in using it. Some women and couples do not use contraception at all, although they could benefit from doing so. They fail to attend either the general practitioner or family planning clinic for advice, but are nevertheless frequent attenders at the surgery for various physical ailments of themselves or their children. Such women or their children are often involved with the social services, and may have children on the non-accidental injury or sexual abuse register. They tend to be labelled as feckless and inadequate, or as 'poorly motivated'. They form the bulk of the work of a domiciliary family planning service, and some of the insights gained in working with them will be discussed later in this chapter.

PRESSURES ON THE DOCTOR

It is perhaps inevitable that the doctor identifies or becomes identified with the medical methods of contraception so that when they are rejected he or she feels rejected too. This can lead to a feeling of uselessness and inadequacy with a sense that there is nothing to offer the patient. In this situation there is a risk of a retaliatory response, either dismissing the patient or attempting to impose a method against her wishes. In that case contraceptive pills are likely to be lost, intrauterine devices pulled out or the patient fails to return.

In these days of clinical audit, when successful contraceptive practice is measured against a fall in the number of terminations, the doctor may feel that all unintended pregnancies must be stopped. Acceptance that not all such pregnancies can be prevented nor every child a wanted one is something the doctor will need to come to terms with. Helping a woman to delay her next child by a few months may be a major achievement, especially if she is struggling with serious internal conflicts or a chaotic lifestyle. Taking time to create a relationship of trust and understanding, rather than one of nonproductive authoritarianism, may well pay dividends in the long run, and the doctor should not feel too much of a failure if there are some contraceptive mishaps along the way.

A common human tendency is to project negative feelings outwards, often onto those who are seen to be in authority. The contraceptive doctor may be the recipient of negative projections when he is seen as the agent of social control, preventing what comes naturally and making value judgements about the reproductive behaviour of others, 'stopping all the lovely babies' as one woman put it. Alternatively, the doctor can be blamed when medical methods fail, especially when the patient has wanted the doctor to take control, and to somehow save her from her own muddle and failure.

The conflict within the individual, presenting as a contraceptive difficulty, may turn into a kind of fight between the patient and the doctor. The patient takes up an extreme position and somehow forces the doctor to take an opposing one. If the doctor can recognize that such a fight is taking place and remember that it is a product of the internal problem (no easy task in the middle of a fight!) some understanding and resolution may be possible. Thus the doctor might say, 'You know, I've been wondering whether this argument we seem to have got into is something to do with different parts of you disagreeing. There seems to be that part of you saying you don't want to get pregnant struggling with the part of you that does, so that on the one hand you do want a reliable method of contraception while at the same time anything I offer is rejected.' This may free the woman to explore her dilemma more openly with herself.

THE IMPORTANCE OF MOTHERS

Girls whose own mothering has been inadequate may be very uncertain of themselves and of their sexual identity. They may have particular fears about the effect of contraception on their fertility, and they may need to establish their femininity by becoming pregnant. For some girls, once pregnancy is confirmed and the reality of coping with a baby is faced, abortion may be requested. For others, having a baby not only establishes their identity but increases their self-worth by providing someone of their own to love. Girls who have been in the care of the local authority are especially vulnerable in this respect.

> Miss C. became pregnant when she was 15 years old. She had been very disruptive at school and the staff were concerned about her home situation. Miss C. had an abortion under pressure from her mother. Attempts to get her to take the oral contraceptive pill failed and eventually she became pregnant again. This time she ran away from home determined to have the baby. She herself had been born out of wedlock and did not know her father. She had been cared for by various relatives. Miss C. felt unloved and unwanted. At 14 she had been reunited with her mother but had to face competition with a younger brother on whom the mother doted. It was perhaps not surprising that Miss C. wanted a baby, someone of her own to love and to love her.

Getting pregnant and having a baby is at some level both identifying with one's own mother and also rivalling her. This can cause anxiety, both for having the temerity to attempt such competition, and also from fear of an envious attack from mother. There may be a wish to triumph over mother, to outdo her or the siblings. There may be the idealization of motherhood with consequent fear of not being so good at the job as mother had been.

Mrs D. aged 21 years had produced four children in as many years. She was a loving mother but exhausted. She seemed set to follow her mother's pattern of having 14 children. Several of these children, including herself, had been in the care of the local authority from time to time, a fact that Mrs D. sometimes remembered and sometimes seemed to choose to forget. She decided to try the intrauterine device but it became increasingly evident with each meeting that a tremendous struggle was going on inside her as shown by her complaints about contraception and her feelings about the doctor (female) which were sometimes hostile and sometimes friendly. On the latter occasions she would express great interest and curiosity in family planning work. The doctor then felt like a warm supportive mother. When Mrs D. was hostile, the doctor felt like a baby-hater out to prevent Mrs D. and all other women from having all the babies she and they longed to have.

At one visit, Mrs D. yet again voiced her anxiety about the harm that the intrauterine device was doing to her insides. The doctor decided to take the bull by the horns and told her about the way she made her feel and wondered if this reflected the way she was feeling. Mrs D. then began talking about her mother who made her feel that having babies was a normal, natural thing to do and that they should not be prevented. However, she also knew that her mother had found it very difficult to look after all her children (though this was usually blamed on their father). Admitting all this made her feel she was being critical of her mother and she hated doing it. The doctor said she did not have to be like or unlike her mother, she could be herself. They agreed that it was obvious that she loved her children but knew she did not have endless patience or energy, and that what could be managed with four children could not be with 14. This seemed to free her in some way and there were no further complaints with the coil.

The case of Mrs D. shows how inevitable and necessary it is for the doctor to become 'entangled' in the patient's problem, allowing herself to feel in response to the patient, as this provides valuable clues to what is really going on in the patient's mind. The doctor must be aware of what she herself feels in order to be able to use the feelings to help the patient to understand herself. In this case the contradictory feelings in the doctor, of being a warm supportive mother and yet also a destructive baby-hater, accurately mirrored the patient's conflict in relation to her mother and babies.

THE FEELING BEHIND THE SYMPTOM

Women using contraception tend to blame the method for many symptoms that are clearly not related in any medical way. If simple explanation does not reassure the woman, it is important to listen further to try and understand what is going on in her mind.

Mrs E., a regular clinic attender for years, came to the clinic one evening in a state of agitation quite unlike her usual self. She had found a lump on her cervix and was sure it had been caused by the contraceptive pill. The doctor examined her and found a small nabothian follicle and tried but failed to reassure the patient, who became more agitated and angry, convinced that the doctor had missed something. The doctor collected her wits and managed not to respond defensively, saying quietly, 'I think I am missing something; you are not your usual self. Has something happened?' At this point Mrs E. burst into tears and said that her marriage had broken up after 10 years and her family were furious with her. They had been convinced that she and her husband were the ideal couple, and she too had thought that she had the perfect marriage. Childless by choice, they were both highly successful in their jobs and owned their own house. However, she had found someone at work and realized that she could enjoy life in a way she had been unable to do in her marriage. She felt guilty about her husband, who ostensibly had done nothing wrong other than be predictable. She had also discovered to her surprise that she now passionately wanted a baby with her new partner. She thought that the lump on her cervix would prevent her getting pregnant and that it was a punishment for being happy at the expense of another.

Shame and guilt are important emotions in contraceptive practice and are often related to past sexual relationships and behaviour. A previous unintended pregnancy and abortion do not necessarily lead to more careful use of contraception, as there may be an unconscious wish to deny what happened and to get pregnant again to make some kind of reparation.

A request for termination can be seen as a symptom, and it is important to try to help the woman to understand the underlying feelings. If she is punishing herself for previous sexual behaviour, failure to explore and understand what is going on may prevent her from taking proper responsibility in her future sexual life. There can also be other even deeper psychological reasons for the request. What, apart from the fetus, is she aborting and why? Perhaps she is aborting her potential to become a mother, fearful of rivalling her mother, as has been mentioned before. Or she may be aborting that fragile, despised baby part of herself deep inside. What does the fetus mean to her? Is it perhaps felt as a kind of parasite, feeding on her and preventing her from growing to her own full potential? It may not be possible for the doctor or nurse without psychotherapeutic training to uncover such feelings, but they need to be born in mind when repeated requests for termination seem inexplicable.

Other symptoms that may hide complicated and ambivalent feelings include overt sexual complaints such as loss of libido. If the patient is taking the oral contraceptive pill the complaint can present a complex problem. While it is possible that the Pill reduces libido, changing the type of Pill or indeed the method of contraception does not often solve the difficulty. The complaint may be due to several factors. The Pill is sometimes regarded as too safe in preventing pregnancy, so that the element of danger and risk-taking is missing. The woman may feel controlled by the Pill, her natural hormones being supplanted. She may believe that if it was not for the Pill she could refuse sex. Unacknowledged problems in the relationship such as anger and resentment that cannot be expressed openly can lead to avoidance of sex, and the Pill can then be blamed making the problem a medical one for doctors to solve.

CONFLICT IN RELATIONSHIPS

Some women are faced with choices that they find very hard to make consciously, and they may then begin to use their contraceptives erratically as though they hope that fate may somehow make decisions for them.

> Miss F. was a 19-year-old who had a steady partner. The relationship had lasted several years and she had taken the Pill regularly with no problems. She felt the relationship was important to her, but she had now gained a university place which would mean moving away from home and from her partner. She felt torn in two, pleased to have a university place but fearful that going away would end the relationship. She began forgetting to take her contraceptive pills and the inevitable happened and she became pregnant. Paradoxically perhaps, this enabled her to make her choice. She now realized that she did not want a baby and realized how resentful she would feel if she did not go to university. She had an abortion and went to university.

The stability and quality of many relationships can determine whether contraception is used and which partner uses it. Where there is trust and openness in the relationship, contraception can be accepted more readily, though there may be resentment that it is needed and a dislike of the actual methods. When there is change in the relationship or when it is unstable, especially at the beginning or the end, contraception may not be used or, if it is, the use is often erratic.

The sexual relationship may be for mutual pleasure and joy, but it can be used to control, dominate or compensate for feelings of inadequacy. By not using contraception there may be an unconscious wish to control or limit the partner's sexual activity. Resentment or envy of the other's sexual enjoyment can also lead to a more overt expression of non-use of contraception exemplified by the phrase, 'Well, why should I take the Pill (with all its dangers) when he is the one who gets the pleasure?'

Allowing a pregnancy to happen by using contraception erratically can be a way of testing the relationship and holding on to a partner. If only one of the partners wants a pregnancy, methods may be sabotaged. Pregnancy can be used to control the woman, especially if there is violence in the relationship. A man who is adamant that his woman's place is in the home may fear loss of control if he does not keep her constantly pregnant. Sometimes cultural and religious views can be called upon to defend the man's position.

> Mr G., an unemployed partially sighted Bangladeshi man, is the father of 11 children and the grandfather of five. Initially, he seemed to accept the fact that his wife was receiving contraceptive advice. He spoke good English although his wife did not. A linkworker was brought in to help interpret. The Pill was chosen and the wife beamed her approval. All went well for about a year but then Mr G. forbade his wife to take it any more insisting that she have another baby as their Moslem religion instructed. It appeared that Mrs G. had no say in the matter and went on to have her twelfth child at the age of 42 years. At her postnatal visit she looked tired and defeated, but Mr G. beamed in triumph and refused to allow his wife to use contraception. The doctor felt angry and frustrated but nothing could be done.

It seems that in this marriage Mr G. felt that his authority was being threatened, perhaps because he was no longer the wage earner, and perhaps as a result of his sense of not being fully in control because of his poor vision. The only way he seemed able to reassert his position was by the use of his fertility.

CARING FOR THE POORLY MOTIVATED

It is not easy to provide care for those who are not well motivated to use contraception, and the way it is done can be a contentious issue. Anxieties may be raised about eugenic control, for instance that one is stopping the poor from breeding, or making value judgements about the behaviour of others and imposing foreign values on them.

Conflict between professional carers is often engineered unconsciously and sustained by the woman or couple concerned. Differing views between doctors and social workers, or between two doctors trying to help the family, can become polarized. 'Splitting' into good and bad is a common phenomenon when working with disadvantaged and deprived families. Sometimes it is the social worker who is good, trying to save the family, while the doctor or health visitor is seen as bad. These positions can alternate, with the social worker regarded as being bad when children are taken into care. It often seems as if professional workers are put into the roles of mother, who is seen as kind, indulgent and nurturing, and father, who is stern and expects achievements. These stereotyped figures then fight over what is best for their 'children'. Indeed, it is not uncommon to hear professionals talking about 'my patients, my clients, my families' as if they were their children. Such unconscious rivalry needs to be openly recognized and acknowledged so that carers can co-operate for the benefit of these families.

Conflict is not the only emotion that gets projected into those who are trying to help. The apathy and fatalism that such families generate can also overtake the professional worker. It may then be decided that nothing can be done, apart from dream about some kind of Utopian solution and, like the family itself, the worker may lurch from crisis to crisis. Debts accumulate, electricity and gas are cut off, children do not attend school and may be neglected or abused. Against this background, talk about contraception can be seen by the woman in a negative way as if it is being advocated in order to control rather than to empower her. Where the emphasis is on trying to change social conditions the subject of contraception can be overlooked, yet the failure to raise the issue and give a realistic appraisal of risks and benefits actually denies people freedom of choice.

How have the negative feelings towards contraception come about in these families? Often both the women and men have grown up feeling that the world is against them. Unloved and rejected by their own parents, lacking self-esteem, feeling powerless to influence their destiny, they live from day to day, unable to plan for the future because there is no belief in a tomorrow. Impulsive behaviour and the seeking of instant gratification are natural results. Feeling as they do, undervalued by society, there is a sense that at least they can have babies. Children can take on the role, as in the case of Mrs A. (p. 4), of a bastion against a hostile world. A baby represents a new beginning, new hope and excitement in an otherwise unfulfilling life. The baby can represent something good that can be produced from what may be thought of as bad sex, for such a woman often has a history of sexual abuse in her own childhood.

Pregnancy itself compensates for feelings of inner emptiness, literally filling the woman with new life. Women who experience this emptiness often feel depleted after childbirth and may be anxious to get pregnant again soon afterwards, resenting any discussion of contraception. The baby can also represent one's own baby self to love in a way that one was not loved. Being a mother enhances status and although mothers are not necessarily treated well, they are regarded as good. Children can counteract boredom and loneliness, providing interest and entertainment, and can satisfy the need to be needed. They can compensate for a lack of material possessions and give a sense of potency: 'Something new created in a material world,' as one unemployed and destitute young man put it when he was asked how he felt about the pregnancy of his girlfriend.

Men who feel inadequate, and who are unable to compete with their peers because of lack of skills and training, may put great emphasis on their ability to get their partners pregnant, some talking of their plans to have a football team. Condoms are mocked; they split and tear and cannot hold back their powerful sperm. Sometimes it seems that there is a continuous battle being waged between the sperm and egg on one side, and the contraceptive methods on the other. 'If you're meant to have a lot of kids then even that Pill can't stop you,' said one woman who helped the process by forgetting a few Pills. Thus masculinity and femininity are often defined in a stereotypical way firmly linked to the ability to have children.

Parenthood is often idealized in an attempt to give children what the parents themselves did not have. The problem lies not in the intentions, which are often very well meaning, but in not being able to address the real needs of their children. Sometimes the children are expected to parent the parents, and are denied their own childhood. In other families any form of separation – weaning, walking, the negative phase of 'the terrible twos' – is experienced by the parents as rejection, and is resisted. A replacement may be sought by having another baby. As one mother of five children put it, she wanted another now her youngest was four because he no longer needed her; he could walk and talk. Being a separate individual with different needs in such families is felt to be too threatening, and importance is given to being the same, of one mind. Family therapists have described these families as emotionally enmeshed.

The impression may have been given that nothing can be done for such families. While this is true for some, it is not for all provided that a trusting, reliable and supportive relationship can be created between the doctor and/or nurse and the patient. However, it can take many years to establish such a relationship, and the professional worker will often be tested to see if he or she really is concerned. This testing can take several forms. In domiciliary family planning, it can mean being out when the doctor calls, complaining about the methods, forgetting to take Pills or to follow advice and so on. Sometimes the testing is to do with control and limits, particularly with some teenage mothers who both want and resent control. Feelings tend to be acted on rather than thought about. The task facing the professional is to survive, not retaliate and to think about the behaviour even when caught up in it. Sharing understanding of the behaviour and the unconscious need for it with the patient can enable her to be more aware of what she is doing. Only then can old patterns be broken.

Mrs H., 24 years old and mother of four children born in five years, was referred for domiciliary family planning. Though her husband worked as a carpenter, the family was in debt and social services were involved. At the first visit Mrs H. gave the impression of someone without any cares. She opted for the Pill, though regularly complained about it, and it was changed twice with no improvement. When the last baby was a year old she left home briefly, significantly when her social worker, to whom she had become very attached, left and was replaced by a new one. When next seen by the family planning doctor she made various derogatory remarks about the new worker. The doctor responded to this by saying it took time to get used to a new person and she must feel sad about the other one leaving. This allowed her to cry, although she did not say much.

By this time Mrs H. had stopped taking the Pill as she said it made her depressed. Soon she left home again, returning pregnant a few months later. While discussing what she wanted to do she began to talk about her own childhood, when *her* mother had often left home, eventually for good when Mrs H. was 11 years old. She and her seven brothers had been put into care. She described her father as strict and hard working, but she was fond of him. This discussion seemed to help her to decide to have an abortion, and this was arranged. At the follow-up visit she recalled her mother trying to perform an abortion on herself with soap and water. This seemed an obvious reference to herself and her own abortion, and perhaps a need to be punished, as she admitted she expected it to be painful. Contraception was discussed with the couple and, despite the misgivings of the doctor and the social worker, Mr H. decided to have a vasectomy.

A year later Mrs H. recontacted the domiciliary service. She had left her husband, had a new partner and was five months pregnant. She decided to keep the baby, but felt guilty as the youngest child was still in care, and she was ashamed to tell her social worker. The doctor encouraged her to do so, and reassured her that no one would force her to have an abortion against her will.

After the birth of this fifth baby her chaotic lifestyle continued. She decided to have the fourth child adopted, and the new baby was in and out of care. During a number of visits the domiciliary doctor learnt that the boyfriend was often violent but Mrs H. felt that she deserved it and that her husband had been too soft. However, she liked men to take her out and give her a good time. The doctor suggested that there seemed to be a contradiction here, wanting a good time and then needing to be punished for it. She agreed laughingly. Eventually she became pregnant again, but this time she opted for sterilization at the time of abortion. When last seen the boyfriend had finally left, Mrs H. had got her three older children with her and was expecting the baby to be returned when he was three years old. Her husband visited her and the children regularly.

Mrs H.'s unpredictable behaviour resulted from her conflict between the wish for a stable life and motherhood and the desire for a good time. She had no model of a stable mother hence her distress and anger when her first social worker left. Hurt and rejected by her mother, she nevertheless envied her apparent free-dom and gaiety. She loved her father but also despised him for being unable to control her mother. These feelings were later trans-ferred to her husband. Without inner control she looked to others for control, but then found difficulty in accepting it. Her very inadequacy as a mother made her get pregnant in the hope that she could prove she was different from her mother. However, each time she found the demands of babies and small children too great.

In this case a measure of understanding about the unconscious forces underlying Mrs H.'s actions, and close co-operation between the doctor and social worker, allowed a consistent approach, and prevented the conflict about control being acted out between those who were trying to help.

Sustained support from the same workers over a considerable time is needed for such women until they can take the responsi-bility for contraception themselves. It is essential for the woman to be supported in her choice of method so that she can learn about her own limitations in using it. Eventually she may come to accept that outside control – in the form of sterilization – is the answer, but this can be done only when the woman herself wants it and should never be imposed.

CONCLUSION

The decision to use contraception or to have a baby always involves ambivalent feelings, which are often based on unconscious factors. It is essential for the doctor to get 'enmeshed' with the patient during the consultation. Understanding of what is happening inside the patient can then be obtained and shared. She can then take more conscious control and make more sensible decisions for herself. Whatever the age of the woman or the couple, and in whatever setting the contraceptive advice is being given, these matters will have to be considered if the patient is to receive adequate care.

REFERENCES

Neumann, E. (1955) *The Great Mother*, Bollingen Series, Princeton.
United Nations (1990) *Population and Human Rights*, United Nations, New
York, p. 41.

2

The method and its meaning

Merryl Roberts

SUMMARY

- Using nothing
- Barriers – 'Now it's your turn'
- What about the mess?
- The power of the Pill
- The coil – balancing risks and benefits
- The injection – out of sight, out of mind
- Sterilization – the final solution

The choice of which, if any, form of contraception to use is one of the most intimate decisions a man and woman can make. The title of this book, *Contraceptive Care: Meeting Individual Needs*, draws attention to the contrast between the needs and perceptions of individual health professionals and the individual needs of those they are trying to help. It could be argued that the word 'care' is hardly relevant here, certainly if used in its literal sense of watching over or tending (Hawkins, 1989). Might we be tempted to use this knowledge, this care, to intrude into, even try to control, other people's private sexuality? And yet, modern contraception is complicated, often highly technical and scientific, and our patients do feel the need to seek our advice. Clearly, doctor and patient share the same difficulty when it comes to balancing emotional and physical needs in this field. Patients bring to even the most apparently uncomplicated consultation their own hidden agenda, which doctors and nurses, intent on the rational and scientific aspects of birth control, frequently miss.

To doctors, methods of birth control fall into five main categories: barrier, hormonal, intrauterine devices, sterilization and termination of pregnancy. To patients there are two main divisions: those you can get on with yourself, and those for which you have to involve others, usually doctors or nurses, and therefore lose some privacy and control. The extent to which this external interference is tolerated depends on many factors, some obvious to medical minds, like the absolute desire not to get pregnant now, and others less clear – a fear of using something perceived as unnatural or artificial, for example. Every method has a different meaning for each individual patient.

USING NOTHING

One gulf between perceptions is well illustrated by contrasting the attitudes of doctors and patients towards the simplest of all methods of birth control – nothing. Unfortunately, the consequences of this method frequently require some medical interference at a later date, postcoital contraception or termination, for example. Doctors tend to see patients who use nothing as being ignorant, feckless or even stupid, and are tempted to treat a subsequent request for help in this light. Many patients will agree, in the cold light of the next day or a missed period, hence the amazing number of reported burst sheaths, but, if the real reasons for using no protection at all are not explored, the situation can easily occur again.

Many users of the 'nothing method' are under 16 years of age. It seems to be the policy of our society to emphasize that using contraception is an adult affair. Social concern with the rising tide of teenage pregnancies may be on the increase, but for the young themselves, newspaper headlines blazon adult priorities and moralities. Should parents be told of medical consultations concerning the under-16s, whatever the wishes of the young individual concerned?

The message is clear, sex is private – unless you use birth control.

It is by no means only young people who have difficulty in reconciling the consequences of sexual intercourse with the strong passions and fantasies surrounding the act itself. Sex can be exciting, rebellious, experimental, a rite of passage into a new world. Condoms are perceived as sordid, evidence of prior planning and thus detracting from the romance, a butt of jokes. No amount of worthy sex education can bridge this gap, unless feelings like these are understood. Also, some women hold themselves in such low esteem, consider their sexual selves so worthless, that the only way they can impress or please is to agree to or encourage sexual intercourse. In young women in particular, pregnancy is often the result, leading to repeated requests for terminations.

> She was 16, and making her third request for termination. The first time, she said, her doctor had arranged a termination at the local hospital, the second time, reluctantly, he had tried, but had had to send her up to London. Now, he had said he could no longer help. She sat there, passively, agitated only by the thought that her mother, who had paid for the second termination, would 'kill her'. Had she tried contraception? A tiny shrug. Sometimes, well, not really, she didn't really get on with it. What a problem, thought the doctor, and dumped in my lap! Both the nurse and the doctor felt angry at the girl, wanting to lecture her on her irresponsibility. The extreme passivity of the girl was striking. The only emotion so far had been directed at the mother. Was all this, thought the doctor, an attempt to rival or get back at the mother? 'And Dad?' asked the doctor. The girl froze. 'Which Dad?'' she said, and began to cry. Out came a sad story. Her real father had sexually abused her. Her mother had found out and left him, taking her daughter: 'But, I *missed* my Dad!' she wept. Now, her mother had a new boyfriend. The girl, angry, powerless, and feeling excluded and rejected, sought attention – in the only way she knew best.

Such women perceive themselves as powerless victims. Their anger, in this case towards the mother and so accurately mirrored by the doctors and nurses, produces retaliation and often leads to unconscious self-destructive and self-punishing behaviour.

BARRIERS – 'NOW IT'S YOUR TURN'

For couples who wish to keep details of their sex life private, and yet still want to use contraception, the easiest method is to buy condoms. In family planning clinics, condoms are available free. However, it is striking how few stable couples return for these, preferring the costly anonymity of the chemist's counter. Condoms are generally seen to be man's responsibility, with all the implications this carries in a relationship. Often women, after years of using the Pill or the coil, develop side-effects or anxieties which puzzle the doctor. It may be some time before the doctor realizes the reason for this, and is able to say, 'You seem to feel the time has come to stop taking the Pill?', allowing the woman to admit: 'It's his turn now. I've done my bit.' This statement reveals interesting insights into the way women feel about most female contraceptive methods. There is a sense that the body has been tampered with, an often unconscious intuition that contraception is artificial, and must be disturbing some powerful internal female rhythm. These feelings can be expressed openly when no more children are desired. They seem to be a way of involving the man in future decisions, even passing this burden onto him: 'He's been spoilt long enough!' A simple question, such as, 'How do you think your husband will respond to this?' can be very informative. An indifferent shrug bodes ill for the sexual relationship and may mean that the woman is not only opting out of contraception.

WHAT ABOUT THE MESS?

The sheath can also be considered to be a clean method, in that sperm is not released into the vagina. Some women feel a disgust for this messy, smelly, sperm-filled ejaculate, and they rush to wash the vagina immediately after sex. In this way they state how dirty sex feels to them, as though sperm sullies the vagina, as a rowdy party would untidy the pristine living room. This is a denial of the excitement and loss of control of climax, when warm fluid floods the vagina.

In exactly the opposte way, many women dislike the sheath because they feel that this exciting wetting is missing.

Mrs A. strode into a busy family planning clinic. She had attended some years ago, when she had tried various Pills, expressing dissatisfaction with them all. The notes in the record sheet had become short and brusque, revealing perhaps the atmosphere of the consultations. Eventually, she had just stopped coming. Today she seemed tense and angry. With a frown, she looked at her watch, making the doctor feel guilty, and yet the clinic was not running late. The doctor found that she herself felt rushed and rather irritated.

'I want a health check,' she commanded, forceful and unsmiling. Doctors and nurses are not used to being ordered about in this way; it is easy for hackles to rise and defences to spring up. The doctor felt attacked and was tempted to retaliate, to point out that this was family planning, not a well woman clinic, for example. Instead, she inwardly observed this difficult atmosphere, and wondered what was behind it. 'We haven't seen you for some time,' she commented. Mrs A. shrugged, but remained silent. 'Are you still on the Pill?' 'No,' another shrug, then defiantly, 'We use a sheath.' The tension level in the room rose. 'Look, I've come for a health check – that's all!' The doctor thought to herself, 'Contraception produces tension, but is not to be discussed.' She changed tack. 'Of course we will examine you. Have you been having any problems?' Immediately, the reply shot back, 'No.' Another glare at the watch. The doctor sat back and waited, refusing to be bounced into this checkup, realizing that, so far, she had been doing the work here. Now she let the patient decide how to continue.

Silence. In the background, the practice nurse looked at her watch. 'My husband and I are no longer together.' Mrs A. looked quickly at the doctor, and then back at her watch. 'I've got a new bloke . . . don't know why . . . just felt I ought to have a check-up . . . ' Suddenly, the defences were lower, and Mrs A. was able to talk about the new man in her life. 'He's smashing, really nice

. . . [another anxious sideways look] but . . . well . . . he don't really get on with the sheath, says he never had to use it with his 'ex'. But, there's no way I am going back on those Pills!' 'Why don't we get on with the check-up,' said the doctor. 'We can talk about it then.'

Behind the screen, although the examination continued as requested, the talk was all of contraception. She had hated the Pill, well, to be fair, her 'ex' was an alcoholic, had wanted sex when fairly drunk, incapable of it later. 'Every time I took that Pill, I felt sick.' The oral contraceptive pill had equalled anger and humiliation. 'When I left him, I said, never, never again.' The doctor commented that the anger at the husband had turned into anger at the Pill, and wondered if it was only the new partner who did not like the sheath. Was sex OK now? Mrs A. blushed. 'Smashing,' she said, in an embarrassed way. 'But it is true, neither of us like the sheath. It seems . . . a bit cold, really.' (The pelvic examination was normal, and Mrs A. had been completely relaxed. It was warm and intimate behind the screen.) Had she thought of the cap? 'It had been discussed, originally, but . . . wasn't it too messy?' 'Well,' said the doctor, 'so was sex, come to that.' Both laughed. A cap was fitted, she took it out, put it in again, 'It's perfect,' she said. 'I like to be able to do it, and I know he will be pleased. Who would have believed it? Fancy that!'

A cheerful, sexy lady left the room. The doctor looked back at her old notes: 'Cap discussed. Positively rejected.'

Initial reaction to the diaphragm or cap is frequently to feel that it is too messy or too much trouble. It is easy for health professionals to forget the taboos which surround touching one's own genitalia, or at least, admitting to doing so. Ignorance or fantasies about the vagina and womb can lead to worries about the cap getting lost inside the body. The sight of a cap, small and neat to doctors, can be shocking to a woman who imagines her vagina to be the size and shape of a tampon applicator. Spermicide cream, so reminiscent of male ejaculate, can unearth feelings that sexual intercourse is untidy and even disgusting, or too exciting to discuss with this nice doctor. This feeling that the cap is messy as a method is linked to the mess of female sexual arousal (Tunnadine, 1992). In the case of Mrs A., once she was in a sexually happy relationship, such a link made the cap more acceptable. Sometimes all these feelings can be barriers not only to using the cap, but they can also prevent full sexual enjoyment, and the consultation offers a good opportunity to widen the discussion beyond just contraception. The woman who gazes with horror at a cap, or shudders with disgust, or says it makes her feel sick is also describing her feelings about her vagina, and may have sexual problems. A sensitive doctor may be able to help a woman who is uneasy about her vagina to feel comfortable and secure, at ease with herself physically and emotionally, able to insert a cap with confidence. The woman who chooses a cap is often concerned that methods seen as artificial, such as the Pill, will damage her body, and in contrast she is usually aware of the protection against disease that the diaphragm gives to the cervix. This sense of safekeeping or guarding of the womb is a common, if rarely expressed, feeling. She also enjoys using a method which is totally in her control, to use when and if she needs it.

THE POWER OF THE PILL

The oral contraceptive pill is one of the most important medical advances of this century. It has given women almost complete control over their fertility. It controls menorrhagia and dysmenorrhoea, protects the ovaries and stops the pain of endometriosis. The new lipid-friendly Pills have been shown to be remarkably safe in women who do not smoke. And yet, it is the cause of great anxiety to many women, who are full of worried questions about the perceived harm it is doing to their bodies. Does the Pill cause cancer? When should they have a break from it? Will it make them infertile? Does it make you fat? It is easy to blame all this on the media and bad publicity, but how true is that? Some women worry more than others, and this seems to have no connection with age, intelligence or education. Why should this be?

The Pill has to be obtained on prescription from doctors. Patients clearly differentiate between this and whatever they can buy over the counter. For example, antibiotics are widely perceived to be more dangerous and give more side-effects than aspirin. Perhaps a medication so powerful it needs the sanction of a prescription will always be seen as potentially harmful. Certainly, the necessity of seeing a doctor or nurse disempowers the patient as far as contraception is concerned. This is the case for 'de-doctoring' the Pill, allowing it to be bought at will. Those against point out that it is essential that the low-dose pills be taken correctly, that regular checks are necessary and so on. Can it be that doctors are resisting losing this power?

Taking a tablet by mouth dissociates contraception from sexual activity. In fact, many women who cannot allow penetrative sex (non-consummation), but have not been able to seek help, keep on taking the Pill for years. They attend for repeat prescriptions, but always have excellent reasons for avoiding vaginal examinations. This public show of sexuality, attending a family planning clinic, picking up prescriptions, even taking the Pill daily, contrasts starkly with the terrified vaginismus if a pelvic examination, or intercourse, is attempted. Here, taking the Pill has been used as part of a fantasy of normality. The true nature of the sexual problem is often discovered only when a routine smear is attempted. In a different way, couples who value the spontaneity of love-making possible when taking the Pill, are also using a normality fantasy, that is, a method which allows them to pretend there is no need for contraception. Here, the Pill equals freedom from unwanted consequences – a concept popular in the 1970s, perhaps less so in the decade of acquired immune deficiency syndrome (AIDS).

The most immediate and obvious effect of taking the combined Pill is the effect on the menstrual cycle – the actual contraceptive effect is something that does *not* happen. The regularizing and controlling of periods reinforces a view that normality equals a 28-day cycle, that menstruation is unpleasant and the less blood loss the better. However, many women have very positive feelings about menstruation, and take deep, if unconscious, comfort in their body's response to the regular rhythm of the hormonal cycle. To them this monthly bleed is a reassertion of their female powers, a reminder of their ability to conceive and bear a child, even if intellectually a child is unwanted now. The light, exactly regular bleeds of oral contraception trouble such women, although this unease is rarely articulated or even understood.

Mrs B. had happily used the cap, until she became pregnant while doing so. Following the birth, she had an intra-uterine device (IUD) inserted. All was well, until she found herself pregnant again. This new baby, although

deeply loved, increased the financial anxiety of the household, and she and her husband decided that only the Pill
offered them the protection from pregnancy they needed
at the moment. Over the following six months she
changed her Pill frequently, always for the same, vague
reasons: 'I just don't feel me.' or 'I feel tired.' Finally,
she came to see her doctor in tears: 'I've gone right off
sex – I can't bear him to touch me.' At first the doctor
had several good ideas: something to do with coping
with the two small babies perhaps, financial worries or
problems with the husband? All drew a blank, and the
doctor stopped being so clever, and listened to what Mrs
B. wept out. 'It's these periods, for a start, so short –
I'm sure I am not getting a good clear out. What is happening to all the blood that normally comes away? It must
go somewhere. And all those eggs still in the ovaries,
it doesn't seem right. Before I always knew where I was,
I knew when I was going to have a period, and felt so
much lighter afterwards. It just doesn't happen now.'
She felt bereft, she had lost something ill understood but
immensely important to her. After discussion she
stopped taking the Pill, and returned to her normal self.

The Pill is a very powerful contraceptive; taken correctly the chances
of pregnancy are small. This is a great benefit to women, but it is
also a double-edged sword. The desire to become pregnant is not
always an entirely intellectual and rational emotion, and many women
enjoy the element of risk inherent in other, less safe methods. The
very effectiveness of the Pill can trap her, she feels taken over,
becomes angry at this, and this anger is easily transferred to sex itself,
causing frigidity. Sometimes, there is a cogent and usually unconscious
feeling that this total control is cheating nature, that nature will get
its own back in some unspecified way, and no amount of scientific
explanation of the overall benefits of oral contraception will alter this.
Whatever the reasons for unease at taking the Pill, the result is often
that the women forgets to do so, or develops a series of problems
necessitating frequent changes of Pill. She is signalling that the
method, although extremely effective as a form of contraceptive, is
wrong for her. Exploration of the hidden reasons for these anxieties
help her to decide on the method which is best.

THE COIL – BALANCING RISKS AND BENEFITS

It is common for the coil (intrauterine contraceptive device, or IUCD) to be chosen by the woman after all other methods have been discussed and rejected, for whatever reason. All doctors are familiar with the lady who, sitting back in her chair, looks with a marked lack of enthusiasm at the tiny curl of plastic and copper, and says, dubiously, 'Well, I could give it a go.' By this time, the doctor, for medico-legal reasons, has gone into gruesome detail about possible, horrific sounding side-effects, so it is surprising that women choose it at all. The next, inevitable question is 'Will it hurt?' In other words, the woman is accepting that here she is placing herself directly in the doctor's hands, and is prepared to suffer the pain, vulnerability and humiliation of having a foreign body inserted into her precious womb. What can this method mean?

It is sometimes considered that this is a passive response by the woman, placing the responsibility onto the doctor. It has to be said that, as far as this doctor is concerned, such a feeling is rare. This author is usually more aware of admiration for the sheer courage of a woman prepared to undergo this experience. Why should she choose this method?

Certainly, once inserted, the woman has nothing more to do. Few women even check for the threads of the coil, although all are taught to do so. Most women, after the first few months of anxiety – how can such a tiny thing be effective? Has it got lost? Will the bleeding ever stop? – seem to forget that the coil is there, between periods, anyway. Menstruation is frequently heavy, sometimes painful, sometimes preceded and followed by spotting or a brown discharge. Surprisingly, most women are content to put up with this, it seems to be natural, acceptable. It is a price they are prepared to pay. Indeed, sometimes the heavy bleed is seen as a letting out of bad blood, and therefore a good thing. There are women who are grateful that the long menstruation provides an excellent excuse for avoiding intercourse. Other women may return for a check because of a particularly heavy bleed, but if all is well clinically, they go away cheerfully. It is as though the regular, heavy, monthly bleed is actually reassuring – proof that the coil is there, proof that it, and the women themselves, are working.

This is not a perfect nor a 100% successful method, perhaps easier to cope with because of, not despite, these apparent drawbacks. The risk factor, the possibility of pregnancy, is vital to some women if they are to really enjoy intercourse.

Mrs C. definitely knew that she and her husband did not want any more children. However, she could not contemplate sterilization, for herself or her husband. She cheerfully started taking the Pill, but three months later she was back, looking unhappy. No real problems, except . . . well, she quite liked sex, but . . . she could not come any more. Could it be the Pill? Different contraceptive pills were tried, to no avail. It was decided to try the coil, despite the doctor's worries about the risk of pregnancy. She returned happier, the periods were 'miserable', but sex was good again. The doctor initially thought that this depression of libido was caused by the Pill but Mrs C. confided that she had realized that at the point of orgasm she silently called to her husband, 'Give me a baby . . .' She used this fantasy to release herself sexually, and the very unreliability of the coil was its best point.

The coil has many advantages, once fitted it can be forgotten, and sex can be spontaneous. The method seems more natural as it acts on the uterus, in contrast to the Pill which affects the body generally. There is the possibility of pregnancy: 'I could slip up with the coil and it wouldn't be my fault!', but this risk is not great. The trade-off between heavier menstruation and good protection against pregnancy is one that women can come to terms with easily. Although doctors recommend regular checks, the woman, in contrast to the need to return for new supplies of Pills or spermicide, can avoid the doctor if she has no problems. Once the coil has been inserted, the balance swings back in favour of the couple. Perhaps this is the bargain which makes the fear of insertion worthwhile.

THE INJECTION – OUT OF SIGHT, OUT OF MIND

A woman who dislikes the coil can at least have it taken out. This option is not available with injectable contraceptives; it is just a question of waiting for the effect to wear off. British women strongly dislike injections, but for many the prospect of one injection and no need to see a doctor for three whole months, or indeed do anything else about contraception, is irresistible. For this freedom from medical interference, and the equal freedom of feeling like a 'nothing' user, women will risk irregular menstruation, or even amenorrhoea. Most of these women express few anxieties about the method, their main aim is to get 'the jab', and beat a retreat back to privacy.

Marie was brought, kindly but firmly, to the clinic by her health visitor. She was accompanied by four tiny, smiling and scrupulously clean children. Marie lived in a travellers' encampment, in a small van with her five children, her husband and his elderly mother. Her last pregnancy (a baby left with mother) had been difficult, and she had been advised not to have any more, for a while anyway. And there the problems started. She would not take the Pill, would not even think of the cap and was horrified at the coil. Her husband considered the sheath unmanly, and she agreed with him. Marie was shy, modest and adamant. The doctor began to probe gently, listening to her, rather than educating or teaching. The Pill was bad for the body, everyone knew that. The cap seemed dirty, and rules in the van were strict about cleanliness, even when getting water was difficult. The coil gave heavy menstruation. Marie looked embarrassed but explained there were strict rules about periods and sex, and this would make things difficult. At the moment her husband was, well, not doing anything, but this was not right. He needed to love her, and she him. Hesitantly, the doctor suggested an injectable contraceptive, explained the problems but expected a refusal. Marie was delighted; one injection and then nothing for three months! But how natural! No amount of talk about side-effects could dent her pleasure.

STERILIZATION – THE FINAL SOLUTION

Sterilization is only for those who are sure that they want no more children. This is the ultimate in medical interference. An operation, sometimes under general anaesthetic, involving deliberate damage to the internal or external genitalia. From this, there is no going back, and all patients are counselled that reversal operations rarely succeed. Some pain and discomfort is to be expected, and even laparoscopic techniques carry a risk of future gynaecological problems. The first decision each couple have to make is, which one for the 'chop'? Even with the most loving, sexually compatible and stable couple, this can be a difficult decision. There is an element of self-sacrifice here, which may be denied, but is present, nevertheless. One will be damaged, deprived of the ability to make a child, and one will not. One will have to come to terms with this personal loss, which is very different to the couple accepting that there will be no more children in this unit. It is common for the after-effects of sterilization to resemble grief, muted and unconscious though this might be. Grief for the damage, for the ending of fertility, for the children who might have been, but now never will be. The aim of sterilization counselling is to help the couple understand these feelings, and to filter out those for whom the decision is pressurized, or ill understood.

A man might agree to a vasectomy under pressure from his wife because she is angry at her years of contraception, and feels it is his turn now. He may even feel he is being sacrificed, but cannot resist without being thought selfish, or because of a strong need to please her. Either might see the sacrifice as a solution to, or a punishment for, a problem which is not directly one of contraception – sexual, marital, financial and so on. In this case, sterilization can be seen as part of a marital battle, and not purely a contraceptive choice.

However, where this method is chosen for good reasons, the balance for the couple is clear. They exchange total medical control of the operation, plus some discomfort, for a future sexual life completely free of any interference from doctors, no matter how well meant or caring.

For both patient and doctor, the choice of contraceptive method is a question of balancing the wanted effects against unwanted ones. For the doctor this may seem a medical decision, but it is far more complex to the user. A desire for privacy, a conscious or unconscious fear of artificial interference and an added zest to sex if a pregnancy is possible, even if not wanted, are rarely discussed in the family planning clinic. For the patient, the need to be in control of one's sexual life is weighed against the undoubted benefits of modern contraception with the consequent medical intrusion. The health professional who understands this hidden agenda can offer care in its true meaning.

REFERENCES

Hawkins, J. (1989), *Oxford Paperback Dictionary*, 3rd edn, Oxford University Press.

Tunnadine, P. (1992) *Insights into Troubled Sexuality*, Chapman & Hall, London.

3

Care of the younger patient

Bozena Davies

SUMMARY

- How they come
- The need for choice
- The method chosen
- The genital examination
- Psychosexual problems in young people
- What about the boys?
- The very young
- The older 'young' patient

How should 'younger' be defined when considering patients seeking contraception? Should it be by chronological age or by sexual and emotional maturity? If the latter is the yardstick, then the younger patient may be 13 or 30. The emotional tasks of adolescence, and the normal ages at which they are accomplished, have been described by Christopher (1992). The degree of emotional maturity, and the speed with which it is reached, varies widely between individuals, so that the professional offering help needs to be constantly aware that a consideration of the actual age of the patient is not enough to understand the emotional, sexual and contraceptive needs and difficulties.

For the main body of this chapter, the younger patient will be taken to mean the teenager or adolescent. Among these, doctors will see very few who are under 15 years old. These very young girls will be dealt with separately at the end of the chapter. It is estimated that 18 000 15-year-old girls took formal advice on contraception in 1990 in England. In total, all those under 16 years comprise less than 4% of the total workload of what is regarded as a young person's clinic in a large city (Brook Advisory Centre, 1990). However, they are an important group, not only in terms of health care in its widest sense, but because they fall into a special category as regards legal and ethical considerations.

The age of consent to sexual intercourse for a girl, at present, is 16 years in Great Britain. It is legally allowable to offer contraceptive advice without parental approval provided the following conditions are met. The doctor must encourage the girl to discuss the matter with her parents if she possibly can, there must be evidence that she is likely to be at risk of pregnancy and she must be mature enough to understand what she is doing. For a fuller discussion of the development of the present legal position, the reader is referred to a useful publication produced by the National Association of Family Planning Doctors (Biddell, 1986), and to the Brook Advisory Centre publication, *Under Sixteens: The Law and Public Policy on Contraception and Abortion in England and Wales* (1993). Doctors in England follow guidelines produced by the General Medical Council (1991a; 1991b), and by the British Medical Association (1988).

Despite the wide variation in sexual and emotional maturity mentioned above, the majority of young people, who are in the throes of separation from parental dependence and embarking on a sexual life of their own, are doing so at a chronological age that lies within the normal limits for the society in which they live. Contact with doctors at this age is rare, so that even without its sexual connotation, the appointment with the doctor is special to the patient. Confidentiality is of paramount importance. Whoever is the first contact, be it a nurse, doctor or social worker (in those few clinics where one is available), a tone needs to be set which will allow the individual time to express needs and wishes. Each patient should be able to sense that this very important step in their life is being treated in confidence, as well as with respect and understanding.

An 18-year-old girl attended a clinic two hours away from her home. A new doctor expressed surprise at the distance she had travelled, noting that she had been attending for four years. 'I like coming here,' the girl said. 'I know I ccould go to a nearer clinic, but I first came here in a state, needing the 'morning-after' pill.'

Her first experience was good, and she found the staff kind and friendly. At that time she had been worried on two counts, the risk of pregnancy and the risks of the Pill. Her mother had frightened her with myths about the Pill causing breast and cervical cancer. She felt that at the clinic her anxieties had been given credence and replaced by information. Four years on she is a happy Pill user who prefers to return for her contraceptive care to the clinic where her first experience, in a crisis, was good. This girl, only 14 years at the time of her first attendance, had achieved a considerable degree of emotional maturity, being able to take responsibility into her own hands and finding the first contraceptive consultation all that she had hoped for.

Younger patients are looking for a friendly place, with an atmosphere that is nonclinical and informal, in which to make their contraceptive consultation. They hope the staff will be welcoming and nonjudgemental, but they also expect them to be well qualified, to have medical expertise and to be professional in their approach. Unfortunately, young people often regard doctors in general as impersonal and uncaring. They are thought to, 'Lay into you and interrogate you'. As one patient said, 'Don't they realize that family planning is not the sort of thing that young people have experienced before and that we need time and understanding?' The ideal doctor is described as one who is friendly and who is prepared to sit and listen. Such qualities are usually seen as more important than the sex of the doctor. However, to those aged under 16 years, the doctor's sex matters more, with nearly nine out of ten girls in this group wanting to see a woman doctor (Allen, 1991).

HOW THEY COME

When they first attend, the majority of teenagers have already been sexually active, for a varying period of time, usually using condoms for contraception, at least on some occasions. They come saying they want a safer method and most are hoping for the combined oral contraceptive (COC). The second commonest group, again sexually active, are happier and more reliable sheath users but have experienced a sheath accident and are attending for emergency contraception. Many of these, after receiving postcoital contraception (PCC), if appropriate, will want to consider a less risky method for the future. 'I don't want to go through that again,' is a commonly heard expression. A smaller number in this category will continue to use the sheath as their sole method of contraception.

Virgins who are in a relationship and expecting to be sexually active often appear to want a particularly reliable method. The words used by this group, 'safer' and 'certain', illuminate the different way they perceive their needs. Such feelings may be a sign of a more mature realization of the outcome of intercourse. Doctors may be particularly worried by these patients because of the fear that providing contraception may encourage them to embark on intercourse before they are ready. Some girls who come for help before starting to have intercourse have thought deeply about the situation and are able to make sensible decisions for themselves. Others come for more dubious motives, such as the need to conform to peer pressure, and later problems may develop if a girl appears to be ambivalent about beginning contraception, as is shown in the case of Miss R. described below.

A smaller number of patients attend after a termination of pregnancy. Some of these have already discussed contraception or indeed have started taking the Pill immediately after their termination. Others have delayed thinking about their needs for a variable length of time. Among these, as also among young mothers, there may be many problems, expressed overtly or covertly. A common finding is that during their recovery, from either a termination or childbirth, they have felt themselves unable or powerless to choose.

An 16-year-old girl, Miss R., with a six-week-old baby came asking for the injection. She looked dull and resigned. The doctor felt hopeless and wondered why this method had been chosen. As the girl talked, the doctor sensed that she had been thought to be irresponsible by those who had looked after her during and after the pregnancy, and therefore only the injectable

contraceptive, medroxyprogesterone, had been discussed postnatally. Given time, she chose the COC and
left, looking quite bright, and saying 'nobody explained
it properly before'.

The vast majority of patients come on their own into the actual
consulting room, though they may have come to the clinic with a
girlfriend. Occasionally, the patient will ask if the friend can come
in with them. The sensitive doctor will make the distinction between
those who are nervous (true fear of the unknown) and those in whom
the need for support may shed light on their emotional maturity. The
boyfriend is also sometimes in the waiting room and may ask to come
in with his partner, or she may ask him to do so. Here again, from
the verbal and nonverbal communication of the two, the doctor will
gain some insight into what the boyfriend's presence might signify.
Is he genuinely offering support in a loving way? Is he concerned
about the perceived risk factors, or has he come for further information about the methods?

The number of boys asking for help for themselves is very small,
in line with the general under-use of contraceptive services by men.
In a given year, the ratio of women to men seeking contraception
(all age groups) in a city is 25:1 (Brook Advisory Centre, 1990).
Efforts are now being made to provide services that are more attractive to men, such as men-only clinics. It is hoped that such clinics
might be able to tackle the problems of contraception and human
immunodeficiency virus (HIV) infection together.

The boys come predominantly for condoms and may be provided
with supplies without seeing the doctor. However, many doctors try
to see them at least once, or make sure that they are offered an
opportunity to come and talk, as a request for sheaths is often a
calling card which they have used in the hope of getting help with
some other anxiety or problem (Hutchinson, 1983). Insistence on
making them see a doctor should be avoided as that could put them
off, but if the clinic staff are sensitive to the unspoken needs of
patients they may be able to offer help themselves, or smooth the
young man's passage to the doctor.

It is always useful to start by seeing people as they wish to be
seen, as individuals, couples or even in more bizarre combinations.

Four young people asked to see the doctor together. One
man, rather older than the others acted as spokesman,

and it quickly became apparent that he was the moving force behind their attendance. After a short while it was possible to split them up into the two couples, and later to see them individually. The older man's own girlfriend felt she was being pressured to go on the Pill because he did not like using sheaths. Personally she had no wish to do so at this stage, and with the support of the doctor she was able to tell her boyfriend how she felt. Giving him an opportunity to air his own views at the beginning appeared to have made it easier for him to accept her ideas, and they were supplied with some more sheaths. Later she returned asking for the Pill, feeling now that she loved him enough to want to do this for him. The other couple had not started to make love and were on an exploratory visit to the clinic, perhaps partly swept along by their friend's need of support. A few months later and they came back on their own and she started the COC.

THE NEED FOR CHOICE

From time to time any doctor offering a contraceptive service, whether in a clinic or in a general practice, will meet patients transferring from other sources of care. The reason usually given is that of convenience, either of time or place, although some young people will express dissatisfaction with their previous care. The dissatisfaction is almost always about attitudes: 'She was very abrupt'; and about not being listened to: 'Surely I should have some say in the matter?' One of the reasons why patients may evoke such responses in those who are genuinely trying to offer care is the unconscious aggression with which they may approach adults whom they see as being in a position of authority. It must be remembered that one of the over-riding emotional tasks at this age is to break away from parental authority and to develop personal standards and ideals (Hinshelwood, 1983).

The doctor who can tolerate a certain amount of aggressive behaviour, recognizing it as a defence against pain and uncertainty, has much to offer the young patient, who is able to test out new ideas with an adult who is not the parent. Such a role may be more difficult for the family doctor, who has often been felt to be a kind of 'super-parent', called in by the real parents at times of illness when they are unable to manage alone. Younger patients often say, 'I've known him all my life, he's like a father: I can't talk to him about sex.' The importance of an alternative source of advice, where the young person can come and go as she (or he) wishes cannot be stressed too highly.

THE METHOD CHOSEN

The COC is the most common form of contraception chosen by the younger patient. In view of this, it merits most attention in this chapter. The doctor looking after this age group has a unique opportunity to get it right at the first consultation as regards absolute and relative contraindications and risk factors. At the same time the first consultation should allow the equally important input from the patient. History-taking may be tedious but gives both patient and doctor time to get used to each other. The doctor certainly becomes aware of the patient's attitudes and no doubt the patient forms an opinion about the doctor during this interchange. In the end it is the young person's perception of the doctor which determines whether the consultation will be useful. The doctor may become aware that thoughts or feelings about the patient are unusual, and this can lead to a study of the doctor–patient relationship which may throw some light on the patient's problems.

History-taking will not be regarded as an interrogation or intrusion if its relevance is explained. To facilitate rapport during history-taking and to avoid misunderstandings, the doctor needs to be specific and wherever possible avoid medical terminology. Thus the words 'clotted or inflamed blood vessels' may replace 'thrombophlebitis'. It is important that words such as 'migraine' should be understood and the details of the symptom explored. It is easier for both patient and doctor to face the idea that the COC is out of the question now and forever if there is a history of focal or crescendo migraine, at the first consultation (Guillebaud, 1985).

If the history is taken thoughtfully, the younger patient perceives that care is being offered and that her needs are respected. In this context, patients in this group may be keen to find out their rubella status, and to discuss their weight and smoking habits *vis-à-vis* the

Pill. The problem of weight gain may be the over-riding anxiety for the patient, and this is an area where her agenda may differ markedly from that of the doctor, who is concerned with the possible presence of pre-existing obesity as a risk factor. As regards diabetes and heart disease, the patients normally understand the need for their consultant physician to be involved in the final decision. If there is any family history suggestive of increased risks, they usually co-operate readily with any blood test thought advisable. With today's focus on prevention and health checks, such patients do not find this alarming. The breast cancer issue is still awaiting clarification but must be discussed, and an informed choice made, to be reviewed in the light of any future evidence.

Having shared their medical, family and menstrual history with the doctor they are not surprised to be asked, 'How long have you been sexually active?' and 'Any problems with sex itself?' Additionally, they see the taking of routine smears as a positive health check. If the sexual history is known and recorded then it is unlikely that a smear will be suggested to a virgin. When the offer of a smear test is refused, it is worth spending sometime looking for the reason behind the refusal. Reasons given can include the rather vague 'I can't be bothered', which may be a sign of a general lack of esteem and self-care, but is more likely to be a way of voicing embarrassment, or even a sign of a phobia of any clinical procedure. An open-ended nonjudgemental enquiry into the difficulty can usually allow the patient to express her fears.

With all young people, indeed with most patients of all ages, the doctor will be considering the question of sexually transmitted disease and how best to introduce the subject. Most doctors encourage the use of condoms for every act of intercourse even if the Pill is also being used, but one has to remember that quite a lot of men have difficulty using them, losing their erection when they try to put them on. The embarrassment so commonly felt about using sheaths can be helped by discussion with nurses or doctors who are not themselves embarrassed. A postal survey of 15 000 women done recently for a woman's magazine found that 25% were so sure of their partner that condoms were never used, and 17% of women said that their partners always used condoms during sex. It is often difficult for the girl to raise the subject with her boyfriend, but the doctor can help by discussing how she might negotiate the matter. Alternatively, if he can be encouraged to come in with her, the tactful doctor can discuss the matter with the couple. Unfortunately, it is often the most responsible boys who pluck up the courage to come to the clinic, and the boyfriends of those girls most at risk are not seen.

Some young women, particularly those who are very health conscious, like the idea of the diaphragm, with 1.6% of new patients and 2.9% of old patients choosing it at the Birmingham Brook Advisory Centre in 1989 to 1990. It does have the advantage of providing some anti-viral effect by means of the spermicide, but as there is not a complete physical barrier to sperm, it does not offer such effective protection to the cervix or against infection. In addition, the failure rate makes it a risky method for those who need the most effective protection against pregnancy, and the lifestyle of many young people does not make the use of a cap very easy. However, the highly motivated couple may be happy to use the diaphragm and the sheath together, thus providing a high degree of protection against both pregnancy and infection.

THE GENITAL EXAMINATION: SMEAR TAKING

An unhurried, gentle approach is valued by this age group during what is often their first genital examination. The doctor should give some thought to minimizing discomfort. Choosing a warm, small speculum for the first smear is one obvious kindness. The question 'Will it hurt?' should alert the doctor to the possiblity that the patient may have some degree of 'dis-ease' with that part of the body, which may present as vaginismus. Allowing time to explore what may be behind a question like that, rather than attempting to reassure or give opinions, may allow the patient to reveal anxieties. More significant in terms of psychosexual problems is repeated procrastination or cancellation of smear appointments. All too often this type of behaviour is seen as irresponsible, when instead it should alert the doctor to the possibility that the patient may have a psychosexual problem. The young patient knows that exposure of this part of the body will expose her sexual difficulty and is fearful (consciously or unconsciously) of doing so.

PSYCHOSEXUAL PROBLEMS IN YOUNG PEOPLE

In a specialist psychosexual clinic, those under 20 years comprise less than 10% of the total workload. However, they are an important group. Some patients in this age group are able to tell their doctor openly about the problem (see Miss A., Chapter 12, p. 181). However, others do not find it easy to raise the subject, and doctors need to be alert to cover problems that may be suggested by a patient's discomfort with her genitals or breasts. Problems that develop in a patient on the Pill may be straightforward physical side-effects, or a covert presentation of a psychosexual difficulty. Many younger patients feel they should report side-effects, more or less obeying the doctor's instructions, whereas older contraceptive pill-users tend to report side-effects that they are worried about. Young patients who develop one side-effect after another, or those who cannot find a method to suit them, should make the doctor particularly alert to the possibility of underlying difficulties. The following case quickly developed a 'thick folder', that sign that general practitioners recognize so well as a warning of possible emotional problems.

Miss R. was 17 when she first attended the clinic and 21 months later had a thick file, having attended 18 times. In retrospect, the professionals should not have been surprised that she wore them down. The counsellor was the first contact and noted that she had been brought/referred by her boyfriend who stayed in the waiting area. The counsellor wrote, 'Has not yet had full intercourse, would like to discuss COC, has steady boyfriend. Will probably have arranged marriage when older and so ambivalent about starting to have sex, will not want future husband to know that she has been sexually active.' A nurse took a history, a doctor saw Miss R. and prescribed the COC.

   Two months later Dr A. saw Miss R. for the first time. Small, dumpy and childlike, she poured forth an amazing torrent of naive and sometimes bizarre questions. 'Was this right, was that right, should he ask her to do this, should it last so long?' Foolishly, Dr A. did not read the counselling notes and tried to deal with these questions as they came, feeling overwhelmed, but unable to interpret to the girl that she, too, was probably feeling overwhelmed by the demands of her boyfriend. Dr A. wrote, 'Examine next time', and fled from the patient feeling exhausted. Interestingly, the girl had also complained of being exhausted.

At the next visit Miss R. had stopped taking the Pill and then started it again, and had many complaints about feeling weak and tired, and having vague aches and pains. Again, she was not examined. During the next year she saw many different members of the clinic staff with complaints about sore breasts, fear of infection, pain in her leg (which could have been a deep vein thrombosis), and continuing anxieties about her parents finding out she was on the Pill, and about her marriage prospects. Finally, one day Dr A. noticed that the boyfriend was always in the waiting room, and was able to lead the patient to a discussion of the question of choice, and the patient's right to say yes or no to sex. This led to further questions about virginity, and the state of her hymen, although again no genital examination.

Following this important consultation her visits to the clinic became less frequent, and later she was able to admit that she was not ready for sex when she started and that she should not have done it. However, there was no discussion of the feelings that led her to start.

This cautionary tale illustrates how a patient's thick folder arises. Such a story should alert the doctor to the probability of a psychosexual problem which has not been resolved. It is interesting that at no time was there any exploration of the girl's own sexual feelings, perhaps because no proper psychosexual vaginal examination had been made, despite various attempts at swab and smear taking, when she was always very tense. Another lesson to be learnt is if there is dissatisfaction with the contraceptive method it is worth referring back to the notes of the very first consultation, for the clues are often there.

THE VERY YOUNG

Very young girls provoke strong reactions in doctors and others, especially if they emphasize their youth by coming to the clinic or surgery in school uniform. They may come on their own, in which case they are usually showing a degree of maturity in taking their own decisions. Often they are brought by someone else, and then the doctor has to try to assess the real needs and wishes of the girl herself.

A 13-year-old girl came to the clinic with her mother. Mother did all the talking, saying that her daughter was in a relationship with a 22-year-old man who had two young children. Mother thought her daughter should go on the Pill as she foresaw intercourse occurring. The doctor felt pity, anger and anxiety as she noticed that the girl was small and thin, her face pinched and hard-looking, trying to look older than her age. The doctor managed to see the girl alone and said, 'I wonder what you expect from this visit?' The girl replied, 'I expect I'll get stuck on the Pill'. This made it easier for the doctor to say what was uppermost in her mind, that the girl had choice. Slowly, as the consultation continued and with the doctor trying to respect the girl's feelings and treat her as a responsible person in her own right, the girl changed, her face softened and she allowed herself to look her age. She said that she did not wish to decide anything that day, and certainly did not want to take any pills.

When a young person is brought to the doctor by someone older, whether parent, teacher, social worker or friend, it can be very helpful if the anxieties of that person can also be examined. When working in a clinic with a social worker it is often possible for her to conduct this interview. In a normal surgery or clinic the doctor will usually have to see both the girl and the accompanying person. It is important that the girl agrees to this and has trust that her confidences will not be broken. She may well be relieved when the worries are eased and some of the pressure is taken off her. Such a dual role can be particularly difficult for the general practitioner with responsibilities to the whole family, and he or she is often grateful to be able to obtain help for the girl from another doctor.

THE OLDER 'YOUNG' PATIENT

Older women who choose to come to a young person's clinic can be viewed as slow developers who are completing the tasks of adolescence late. Often they are only now developing a mature sexual identity, and may be on the brink of making what they hope will be a satisfying heterosexual relationship. They present a different challenge to the doctor. Though adult attitudes prevail during the consultation and history-taking, a larger proportion will conceal psychosexual problems, which may come to light at the genital examination.

Miss C., a 30-year-old patient who was on the Pill, attended the clinic for routine repeat of supplies. She was an attractive woman of eastern origin, who was due for a repeat smear. When the speculum touched the introitus the woman's legs clamped together and her hand came down to push the speculum away. 'I can't,' she said. 'It hurts too much.' The doctor wondered how the previous smear had been managed. 'Oh, I just screwed myself up and let the doctor get on with it, but it was awful and I've put off having another one.' Patient and doctor decided to postpone the smear and talk about the pain. Miss C. seemed happy to stay on the couch and told about her decision not to have sex when her friends first took the plunge. She chose to wait for a special man. When she finally lost her virginity (her words) she was 26 and her first sexual encounter was 'very funny'.

She stayed with her first lover for three years, but now she had a new partner and she was sure he was the right one for her. Sex was fine with him. The doctor wondered out loud how sex was possible in view of her reaction to the speculum and the doctor's fingers. 'Oh, the penis is different – but fingers are forbidden – my partner knows that and is happy to go along with it.' At the next meeting Miss C. confessed that sex with her first lover had always been painful. It seemed that her use of the words 'very funny' was a way of describing the screwing up she had had to do to endure love making as well as smear taking.

During her first tentative self-examination in the doctor's presence she revealed her fantasies about her

vagina. She thought her long painted finger nails would
cut it. Immediately afterwards she started talking about
her mother, not previously mentioned. 'When I was very
young there always seemed to be blood around and lots
of men. I was with her because I hadn't started school.
When I was older she kept going away to have operations, female operations.'

Sharing these feelings about the potential of fingers and instruments
to cut her precious, fragile vagina, and her painful recollections of
her mother, helped Miss C. to sort things out in her mind, and she
found this particularly helpful as she was thinking about having a
baby and had been anxious about all the procedures.

DILEMMAS FOR THE DOCTOR

The provision of the best possible care for young people in today's
society, with pressure towards sexuality coming not just from the
internal forces towards maturity which have always been present,
but also from the peer group and, most strongly, from the media,
is not easy for the professional. There is an over-riding need to
provide the practical help necesssary to reduce the risks in an
atmosphere that is acceptable to the patient, as has been described
in this chapter. Considerable skill is needed to allow the patient to
feel that her sexuality is allowable and valuable, while at the same
time warning her of the health risks.

What, then, of the more general health education that is offered
to other patients? The family planning consultation is seen as an ideal
opportunity to broach such subjects as smoking and obesity, but the
young person may feel such advice to be 'yet another lecture'. If
given unthinkingly, she or he may be antagonized so that they stop
coming for the contraceptive help which is so desperately needed.
However, if given sensitively and at an appropriate time, the assumption that she or he is now grown up enough to want to look after
themselves can enhance self-esteem.

Perhaps the most difficult dilemma for the doctor, as for young
people themselves in the age of AIDS, is to reconcile the strong,
inevitable and healthy emotional and sexual drives, with the possible
risk of serious damage to their health or even death. The equation

is complicated by the feelings of excitement and guilt that are inevitably present at a time of rapid emotional change and growth.

In conclusion, the younger patient, however younger is defined, needs to feel secure in using contraceptive services. Doctors and others providing them can play an important role, not only in helping the young to protect themselves from the unwanted effects of sexual activity, such as pregnancy and infectious diseases, but by providing consistent and concerned care in its widest sense. Such care must be provided by an adult who has respect for the individual whatever their chronological or maturational age, but who can at the same time recognize the conflicts and inconsistencies that are a natural part of adolescence. At a time when conflict with parents is common, an alternative nonjudgemental adult can provide a focus of stability. In particular, such care may help young people to value their sexuality and use it in such a way as to enhance their lives and relationships.

REFERENCES

Allen, I. (1991) *Family Planning and Pregnancy: Counselling Projects for Young People*, PSI Publishing, London.

Biddell, S. (1986) *Children, the Law, Confidentiality and Treatment*, National Association of Family Planning Doctors, 27 Sussex Place, Regents Park, London NW1 4RG.

British Medical Association (1988) *Philosophy and Practice of Medical Ethics*, BMA, London.

Brook Advisory Centre (1990) *Birmingham Brook Advisory Centre Annual Report*, Brook Advisory Centre, London.

Brook Advisory Centre (1993) *Under Sixteens: The Law and Public Policy on Contraception and Abortion in England and Wales*, Brook Education and Publications Unit, London.

Christopher, E. (1992) Adolescent sexuality, in *Psychosexual Medicine: A Study of Underlying Themes* (ed. R. Lincoln), Chapman & Hall, London.

General Medical Council (1991a) *Professional Conduct and Discipline: Fitness to Practice*, GMC, London.

General Medical Council (1991b) *Guidance for Doctors on Professional Confidence*, GMC, London.

Guillebaud, J. (1985) *Questions and Answers in Contraception*, Pitman Press, London.

Hinshelwood, G. (1983) Youth advisory work, in *The Practice of Psychosexual Medicine* (ed. K. Draper), J. Libbey, London.

Hutchinson, F. (1983) Youth advisory work, in *The Practice of Psychosexual Medicine* (ed. K. Draper), J. Libbey, London.

4

The doctor and the unplanned pregnancy

Alessandra Bispham

SUMMARY

- Unplanned or unwanted?
- Ambivalence about pregnancy
- Counselling the patient with the unplanned pregnancy
- Factors in unplanned pregnancy
- The patient who presents late
- How can the doctor with psychosexual training help?
- After an abortion
- If the pregnancy continues

Greater social and medical sophistication in our society has also meant greater involvement between the medical profession and pregnant women. Doctors have become increasingly responsible for the health of the pregnant woman and her unborn child. Laws designed to liberalize abortion have also made doctors more involved with unwanted pregnancies. Throughout the ages and in all societies women have sought to control their own fertility using methods ranging from trying to abort themselves and obtaining an illegal abortion, to infanticide. Although the consequences were sometimes disastrous, it did mean either that women took measures themselves or sought the help of other women. Doctors now have the legal power to terminate a pregnancy and the knowledge to do so safely. If there had been another method of procuring abortion, not requiring medical skill, it is doubtful that doctors would have been so involved. The abortion pill has proved to be a disappointment to women in this way as it still involves medical input. Many women feel that the decision as to what happens to their own body and their own pregnancy should be theirs alone and resent the need to ask doctors for permission to terminate their pregnancies.

The responsibility of dealing with abortion rests uncomfortably on the shoulders of the medical profession. Doctors are trained to preserve life and many feel a moral and ethical objection to terminating it. However, views are often confused and despite vociferous objections to liberal abortion from many in the medical and nursing profession, they themselves have been shown to make good use of the abortion services (Potts, Diggory and Peel, 1977). A further difficulty is that the patient has usually made her own diagnosis and has prescribed her own treatment. Medical training, on the whole, teaches doctors to take a careful history, evaluate the symptoms, make a diagnosis and offer treatment and advice. This may lead to some doctors finding it difficult to be mere technicians, responding to the patient's wishes. Overall, therefore, in dealing with a woman with an unplanned pregnancy, we may end up with a reluctant doctor and a reluctant patient.

UNPLANNED OR UNWANTED?

These terms are often used interchangeably. Unplanned may also mean unwanted. For some women, an unplanned pregnancy may be a very unwelcome intrusion into her life. For others, unplanned pregnancies may not necessarily be unwanted. It is estimated that up to one third of pregnancies may be unplanned (Fleissig, 1991). Some women may go on to term because of moral objections to abortion, but some of these unplanned pregnancies do become very much wanted. Efficient contraception is meant to lead to 'family planning' but we all know plenty of women who look lovingly at their bulging abdomen and say, 'It wasn't planned' Efficient contraception means being able to take responsibility for deciding when to have a baby. To some this means waiting for the right situation in terms of marriage, accommodation, money and career. It also means being able to say to the world that they are now mature enough to become a parent and responsible enough to care for another individual. Some women can allow themselves to have a baby in less than ideal circumstances only by allowing it to be unplanned.

> Miss A. came to the family planning clinic accompanied by her fiancé. She requested a pregnancy test which was positive. The couple came into the office beaming with pleasure. Miss A. had missed a few Pills but they really 'couldn't understand' how she had fallen pregnant. However, they felt sure of parental support and would just hasten their wedding plans. This apparently unplanned pregnancy was obviously not unwanted. The doctor wondered how unplanned this pregnancy was but further discussion at this point seemed irrelevant. The couple wanted the doctor to share in their good news and point them in the direction of antenatal care.

Some very definitely planned pregnancies may turn out to be unwanted. This may be due to a change in circumstances such as deterioration in the relationship, bereavement or redundancy, making the woman feel unable to care for a child or change her objectives. Sometimes a woman may like the idea of becoming pregnant, but once faced with the prospect of having a baby in a few months, she makes a more realistic appraisal of her circumstances.

> Miss B. was a pretty blonde woman who requested abortion. She came to the clinic accompanied by her boyfriend. Immediately, she stated that she did not want an abortion but that *he* did. Her anger was obvious and it seemed he had been brought to the clinic to suffer. She had come off the Pill some months earlier 'to give her body a rest', they had not used contraception and they were both apparently aware of the possible consequences. He went on to say that the relationship had been going through difficulties and he did not feel she was mature enough to look after a baby. She felt she could do so perfectly well if he supported her. They both

realized that they were using this pregnancy to sort out their relationship once and for all. They wanted more time to talk and made another appointment. Miss B. returned alone, looking more composed. Her boyfriend had agreed to her keeping the baby but had placed so many conditions that she felt her life would be intolerable. She wanted an abortion and hoped that one day she would be able to have a baby with someone who was right for her.

Although not consciously sought, this pregnancy was not altogether unplanned. The cracks in the relationship did not really show until the couple had to face this crisis together and their differences became obvious. Miss B. seemed to mature a great deal in the course of a week and moved from blaming him for the abortion to claiming responsibility for her own actions and making her own decisions.

AMBIVALENCE ABOUT PREGNANCY

Most steps forward in life involve giving up some of the old as well as gaining the new, from straightforward events such as changing school or job, to complex maturational stages such as moving from childhood to adulthood. The grief of giving up the old combined with anticipation of the new gives rise to very mixed feelings. Falling pregnant is no different and most women, even when the pregnancy has been planned and wanted, experience times of sadness or fear during their pregnancies, including some of the feelings listed below.

Some *positive* feelings in pregnancy include:

1. Feeling truly feminine;
2. Feeling she has a role in life;
3. Looking forward to something to love and love her;
4. Following in mother's footsteps;
5. A feeling of continuity and eternity;
6. An opportunity to give up an unfulfilling work role and take on a more comfortable domestic one;
7. Approval by family and society.

Some *negative* feelings in pregnancy include:

1. Loss of freedom;
2. Loss of income;

3. Loss of a job, career prospects and status;
4. Fear of losing sex appeal;
5. Making her sexuality public;
6. Feeling she can no longer be a child herself and have to take a responsible role;
7. Fear of being an inadequate mother;
8. Disapproval of family and society.

The particular woman's circumstances, her support network and her own coping mechanisms and ethical framework will influence her decision as to how to proceed with any particular pregnancy.

For some women the factors can be equally balanced, making a decision very difficult.

> Mrs C. is a married woman in her late 30s. Her existing children are growing up a little, she enjoys her independence and plans further education for herself. Although she has always liked the idea of another child, this pregnancy was unplanned (she has an IUCD). She loves babies but also values her newly found independence.

Whatever this woman decides will involve loss, either of a baby or of independence and education. Her age means she feels that another opportunity for a baby or for college may not come along. So this to her is a once-and-for-all decision. In the clinic she was initially very angry and critical of the staff. When this was pointed out to her she could see that she was angry at being pregnant and being placed in this position, and critical of herself for even considering abortion when she had a husband and a home.

Sometimes the ambivalence can be due to a conflict between what the woman wants and what she ought to do. She may be subject to the pressure of others and fear criticism. She may use the abortion clinic for permission to continue with the pregnancy.

> Miss D. was 25 and lived with her boyfriend. She had become pregnant for the second time, having had an abortion at 19. The doctor asked, 'You want an abortion?' She said, 'No, I don't really.' She went on to reel off a list of reasons, many of them financial, as to why she could not have a baby. The doctor pointed out that she had given some very reasonable reasons for requesting abortion but had not said anything about her own

feelings. She continued in the same vein. Recognizing her defences, the doctor tried safer ground and asked how she felt about her previous abortion. She had felt awful afterwards, as she had wanted the baby but could not have it. She was only 19 then. And now? She felt she was the right age but she and her boyfriend were in debt and lived in one room. The doctor said it must be sad to have an abortion when you really want a baby. At this point she burst into tears. She agreed she wanted this baby but felt she could not have it in her present circumstances. She wanted more time to think. She came back a few days later. She had talked to her boyfriend who was delighted at the thought of having a baby, and her parents were going to help out with the money problems.

This woman stated straight away that she did not want an abortion and seemed to be asking for permission to have a baby in her less than perfect circumstances. The doctor acknowledged her very real financial problems but also acknowledged her desire to have a baby.

COUNSELLING THE PATIENT WITH THE UNPLANNED PREGNANCY

There are certain basic differences in counselling a woman with an unplanned pregnancy compared to other counselling situations (Coles, 1983). First, there is a definite time limit. If the woman is contemplating abortion, this is safer and easier if performed before about 12 weeks' gestation. As it can take some time to organize a hospital appointment and a bed, this may result in little time for discussion between diagnosis of the pregnancy and arranging a possible abortion. Sometimes it is better to make the arrangements first and then allow time for counselling, cancelling the appointment later if necessary.

Second, a decision has to be made. One would normally not advise anyone to make an irreversible decision at a time of great stress, yet if the pregnant woman avoids making a decision, a baby will arrive. A further problem is that the doctor has the legal power to agree or disagree to an abortion. Some women may resent this power, or feel they have to give a good enough story to convince the doctor, thereby making it difficult for the doctor to know what they really feel. For this reason, many clinics have nonmedical counsellors. The doctor can diffuse this situation, however, by making it plain at the beginning that he or she is willing to arrange an abortion and then allowing the woman time to discuss her feelings.

Difficulties may arise from the fact that other people are nearly always involved. If a woman is to have a baby, she is likely to become dependent on those around her and the influence of husband, boyfriend or parents is likely to have an important bearing on her decision, even if she chooses in the end to defy them. It is a brave woman indeed who decides to go ahead with a pregnancy totally unsupported, or to have an abortion if that is against the ethics of the people she most loves and would risk losing. Sometimes the picture is so dominated or confused by others that it can be difficult for the woman to sort out her own feelings. This is particularly so with the very young who are still emotionally and physically dependent on their parents, and where the maternal grandmother would often have greatest responsibility in rearing the baby.

> Miss E. was aged 15 and was brought to the clinic by her mother. Mother appeared to be a caring woman who felt it would ruin her daughter's life to have a baby, but she was also concerned because she herself worked full-time and a new baby in the house would be a major disruption. Miss E. sat sullenly and said very little. The doctor asked her mother to leave the room while she examined the patient and tried with little success to find out what her real feelings were. She felt very aware of the generation gap, but an abortion did seem for the best so arrangements were made. Miss E. went in to see the nurses to arrange for her admission. Only then did she say she wanted the baby. The nurse did not book her in but suggested she think things out and come back the following week. She came back this time by herself. She wanted the abortion as she wanted to carry on at school. She had made her own decision now.

Here it was easy for the adults, including the doctor, to take over and decide what was best. It may be that the nurse was less of an authority figure or that by suggesting a date, made the abortion

suddenly seem imminent. However, the nurse let the girl know that
her feelings were important. The outcome was apparently the same
but in the end the girl made her own decision. The prospects for her
emotional adjustment to the abortion (Hutchinson, 1992) and for family harmony seemed greatly improved.

Just as the patient may not make her decision without being
influenced by those around her, neither does the doctor work in isolation. Someone has to carry out the abortion, nurse the patient and,
in the hard-pressed NHS, possibly make the decision as to which
patient is most deserving of a hospital bed. This is obviously easier
in one of the private charitable organizations dedicated to providing
an efficient abortion service. Although no-one may complain at an
extra patient attending the antenatal clinic, an extra abortion on an
operating list may cause exasperation. This author is unfortunately
aware that her counselling is more relaxed when she has plenty of
beds at her disposal than when an admission would involve several
telephone calls. If a woman decides to continue her pregnancy, this
doctor sometimes wonders if she is relieved because she has made
the best decision for her patient, or because she has saved a bed.
One is aware of the warm glow in the staff (and oneself?) whenever
a patient changes her mind and keeps the baby, and how in some
quarters this is regarded as a success. Helping to prevent a woman
from having an abortion she will live to regret is obviously a
favourable outcome but it is a very limited measure of success. A
decision to continue with the pregnancy may not necessarily be in
the woman's best interests.

> Miss F. was a West Indian aged 25. The decision for abor-
> tion had initially seemed straightforward. She intended to
> go to college later that year and a baby would prevent
> this. On the pre-operative round the doctor usually asks
> the patient if she is still sure about going ahead with the
> procedure. To her surprise this patient replied, 'No, I'm not.'
> It was suggested that she should not go ahead that day
> but make another appointment to see the doctor in the
> outpatient clinic. The nursing staff seemed pleased – a
> baby saved and a woman rescued in the nick of time (Potts
> *et al.*, 1977). Miss F. came back the next week. She
> had changed her mind because she had talked to her boy-
> friend who wanted her to have the baby and had made

her feel guilty about having an abortion. However, he was unreliable, beat her up sometimes and was unlikely to modify his own life on the arrival of a baby. College was her chance to get away and make something of herself. She had her abortion the following week.

This woman changed her mind about abortion out of guilt rather than desire to have a baby. The guilt came from her boyfriend who seemed keen to keep her dependent on him. There were also cultural pressures as in her community it was more usual for girls to have babies than to go to college. She wanted to do something for herself and having a baby might have jeopardized her chances. Yet it would have been easy to believe at first that continuing the pregnancy would have been a good outcome.

Bearing in mind all the above difficulties, there are three major components to be considered in counselling a woman with an unplanned pregnancy, not necessarily in this order.

1. Giving accurate information about the options, procedures and relative risks so that the woman can make an informed decision. Despite the fact that abortion is a commonly carried out surgical procedure, it is often not openly discussed. A woman with an unplanned pregnancy may set out with very little accurate knowledge of her options. Much of the information available may be produced by radical pro- or anti-abortion groups carrying strongly emotional overtones. It is important that the woman receives accurate information before making a decision.
2. Allowing the woman the opportunity to explore her feelings about this pregnancy in particular and her fertility in general.
3; Helping the woman reach an understanding as to why she fell pregnant at this particular time. Sometimes this is related to a simple contraceptive failure or mistake (Hutchinson, 1992). She may need help in finding a suitable method of contraception and be given proper instructions as to how to use it. Sometimes the reason for the present pregnancy is more complex, to do with the woman's emotional problems and attitudes to her sexuality. These may need to be understood before she can make use of any contraception offered. She may occasionally need further help from other agencies such as Social Services or psycho-therapy.

The aims of counselling should be to help the woman make her own informed decision about what is best for her, taking into account her external and internal pressures which may influence her so that she can feel more in charge of her decision.

FACTORS IN UNPLANNED PREGNANCY

The Office of Population Censuses and Surveys (OPCS, 1990) figures show that the majority of women having abortions are in their 20s and are single. These women are sexually active and fertile but may not be in a stable relationship, financially secure or established in a career. There is a mismatch between biological maturity and social suitability for parenthood. However, women seeking abortion do span all ages and social situations. The situation is complex (Christopher, 1990) but one can see some broad groups among women seeking abortion as to the factors leading up to the unplanned pregnancy.

Guilt or lack of preparation for sexuality

This is often seen in the very young or women of strong religious beliefs, but can be seen in other women.

> Miss G. is a Moslem woman of 28 years born in this country of Arabic parents. This would be her fourth abortion. On the last occasion she had discontinued the injectable contraceptive, medroxyprogesterone, because her mother had told her it would be harmful. After that she had gone on the Pill but had stopped it for Ramadan. She had no desire for a baby. She was able to talk about her confused feelings about wishing to obey her mother and her religion, but also her desire to be part of western culture and have a sexual life.

Guilt may lead women to feel that sex is something that happens to them rather than something they actively desire and prepare for.

> Mrs H. is a 38-year-old divorcee with a 12-year-old daughter. For the 10 years since her divorce she had worked full-time as a beautician and cared for her daughter, who suffered from asthma. During that time

she had no sexual partner, but then she met a man at a party, was surprised at the intensity of her feelings and ended up pregnant. As she got up on the examination couch she apologised for her unshaved legs saying that she waxed everybody else's legs but never had time to do her own. She was also very concerned that the doctor might find her genitals dirty or smelly. This woman had set aside her own needs in order to look after her daughter. She seemed to feel her own sexuality was something dirty and to be avoided. The fact that her brief time of pleasure had led to an abortion had added to her feelings of self-disgust.

Relationship difficulties

Relationships rarely end neatly and couples may break up and get back together several times in an attempt to confirm their feelings for each other. The woman may give up the Pill in the belief that the relationship is over or perhaps out of anger and pain associated with her sexual life. Lack of sexual pleasure may make a woman less well motivated to cope with the perceived risks and side-effects associated with contraception. Sometimes the pregnancy may be used to test out her relationship, as in the case of Miss B. (p. 51, above). If a woman finds herself pregnant once the relationship has ended, she may decide on abortion not just because of the practical difficulties of single parenthood, but out of a desire to rid herself of everything to do with her former partner.

A chaotic lifestyle

The psychological factors contributing to the chaotic lifestyle of some women have been discussed in Chapter 1. Included in this group are women who are psychiatrically ill, depressed, have drug and alcohol problems, or personality difficulties making it difficult for them to organize their lives. Sometimes women who normally manage their lives well may go through short-term difficulties, for example, a sick child or moving house, so that they are distracted and forgetful.

Attention seeking

Women may become pregnant in an attempt to draw attention to themselves and their difficulties (Blair, 1983).

> Miss I. is 25 but looks younger. She had initially thought of keeping her baby but realized this was only a form of rebellion and not likely to be beneficial to her or the baby. When her boyfriend had found out she was pregnant he had hit her. Her mother had told her to throw the baby out in the rubbish. She felt alone and abused. Her previous boyfriend had been no good and had given her gonorrhoea. She could see all her relationships were harmful to her and talked of her unhappy childhood. A psychotherapy referral was offered and accepted readily.

The reader is referred back to the first case in Chapter 2 for another example of a young woman who repeatedly became pregnant as a way of trying to draw attention to her distress which followed sexual abuse as a child (p. 22).

Women unsure of their femininity and/or fertility

An increasing number of women work outside the home and put off childbearing until a suitable time in their career. After many years of contraception they may feel a sense of panic as the biological clock ticks on. Some women in their lates 20s or early 30s may discontinue the Pill, sometimes just to reassure themselves by seeing their own menstrual cycles, but sometimes pregnancy results. Another group of women may go through a spell of being careless about contraception. After a while they begin to worry about the fact they have not fallen pregnant, even though they did not particularly want a baby. Confirmation of the pregnancy in both cases may bring relief and even a fleeting moment of joy until the woman examines the reality of her situation and realizes that she feels unable to cope with a baby.

THE PATIENT WHO PRESENTS LATE

It is fairly common knowledge that abortions carried out early are relatively easy and carry few risks. Yet a small but steady stream of women present in the mid-trimester requesting abortion. Mid-trimester abortions carry greater physical risk and the woman is more likely to suffer psychological consequences, although this may depend on the method used. A dilation and evacuation under general anaesthetic causes less psychological trauma than a prostaglandin induction (Kaltreider, Goldsmith and Margoles, 1979). For the staff involved, mid-trimester abortions are messy and distasteful. Many NHS clinics refuse to see women over 12 weeks' gestation. Yet this small proportion of women probably require greater skills in surgical technique and counselling, and more emotional support. 'Why did she leave it so late?' is the commonly asked question, carrying the undertone that it was somehow the woman's fault, therefore sparing the health worker any responsibility for helping her.

Some women present late because they genuinely did not believe themselves to be pregnant, often at the extremes of the reproductive age range, or because they have irregular cycles. Some deny the problem until the bulge begins to appear, or hope that they will miscarry. Others sadly may be the victim of a laborious system and unnecessary delays in pregnancy testing and in hospital clinics. Other women are just too inadequate to sort themselves out quickly. A small proportion may delay because of true ambivalence about the pregnancy or perhaps they hope that if they leave it long enough, the doctor will turn down their request for abortion.

HOW CAN THE DOCTOR WITH PSYCHOSEXUAL TRAINING HELP?

Counselling in the case of the unplanned pregnancy has to be brief and to the point. Psychosexual counselling is usually more open ended, allowing patients time to understand their unconscious feelings which may block their fulfilment and allowing a gradual move towards change in attitude. However, psychosexual doctors are trained to listen not only to what is said but what is not said, and to understand what is going on in the consulting room. The specific techniques associated with understanding the doctor–patient relationship and the genital examination can give rapid insight to the patient's feelings which may have nothing to do with a detailed history of her circumstances, as in the case of Miss D. (p. 53) who had enormous financial problems but who still wanted a baby. The genital examination can give the trained doctor an insight into how the woman feels about her sexuality, as in the case of Mrs H. (p. 58), which was important in helping her to understand her feelings about her pregnancy and her contraception. This ability to perform a genital examination in a psychotherapeutic way is a skill which nonmedical counsellors may find difficult to accept or understand.

> Miss J., aged 19, was 17 weeks pregnant. This would be her second abortion. She was very ambivalent about whether she wanted to have a baby or continue with her free, youthful life of going out whenever she felt like it and spending her wages on clothes. She revealed that she had had a lot of physical pain after her previous abortion but denied any emotional pain. She looked away much of the time and conversation was difficult. As the doctor palpated her now large uterus, she said, 'That's my baby. I can take him for walks in the park.'

This young woman was not very articulate. Her pain over her last abortion had been expressed in physical symptoms and only a physical examination enabled her to get in touch with her deepest feelings about this pregnancy.

All counselling should be nonjudgemental. Perhaps it is never more important than in this situation when the patient with an unplanned pregnancy may already be feeling guilty or expecting disapproval. Patients may be distressed, angry or abusive. The feelings may be very intense and directed at clinic staff. It is important to acknowledge and try to understand, rather than react to the behaviour or try to smooth it over. The doctor with psychosexual training is not immune to feeling angry, threatened, sad or at a loss to know what to do, but he or she can sit back, think and listen and use these feelings as evidence of the patient's feelings and by interpretation help them understand their problem.

One learns that all is not what it may initially seem. The patient who is in a great hurry to get everything over and done with, or who asks a lot of technical questions may be afraid of allowing herself to feel. The angry patient may not necessarily be angry at the clinic staff but at herself, her partner or her family, or she may be reacting to an enormous burden of guilt. The bossy patient may feel very vulnerable. The tearful patient may lead one to believe that she is crying over her baby and does not want an abortion. This may be the case, or she may be crying to disarm the doctor, or cover the loss of her own self-esteem. 'I never thought I would end up having an abortion' is a common comment.

The patient who brings someone to the clinic may give valuable information about herself. She may feel too immature or helpless to cope alone, or she may anticipate a battle and bring a friend to fight on her behalf. Partners may come out of true caring but they may also come to make sure she 'gets it done', or they may be dragged along to suffer.

Questions posed by the patient may give clues as to how she feels about herself; for example, a question as to how many women suffer from infertility or have a severe emotional reaction suggests an anxiety that she herself may have anxieties about her own fertility and worries about how she will feel afterwards. It is important to give the patient the facts wherever possible, but also to look at the anxieties underlying the question.

AFTER AN ABORTION

It is wise to offer a post-abortion appointment to check physical and emotional wellbeing and confirm the contraceptive method. Most women will have adjusted well, but about 3% may have emotional problems sufficient to interfere with their lives (Dagg, 1991). These may manifest themselves as depression, anxiety, lack of sleep or psychosexual difficulties: they can be immediate or harboured for years (Conway, Bolt, Cooper *et al.*, 1989). Sometimes the emotional pain can manifest itself as physical pain, resulting in numerous investigations. The fact that some women experience post-abortion difficulties is sometimes used by anti-abortionists as fuel against a liberal abortion law, but the possible emotional trauma of having an unwanted child must be borne in mind (Kaltreider *et al.*, 1979). Sometimes the patient may find it difficult to discuss her feelings after an abortion. She may feel that as she was responsible for this course of action, she should expect no better. Friends and relatives may feel it is something over and done with and therefore not to be discussed. The patient may find her post-abortion check-up a valuable time to discuss her grief and sense of loss.

IF THE PREGNANCY CONTINUES

This may well be a happy event requiring no special support, but an unplanned pregnancy may occcur when a woman feels ill-prepared for parenthood and she may need extra emotional and social support. If she had considered abortion, she may harbour feelings of guilt, sometimes resulting in over-zealous protection of her child. The very factors making her consider abortion may still be present when the child arrives and the practical difficulties will need to be faced.

CONCLUSION

The patient with an unplanned pregnancy may present with many conflicting emotional needs, which require rapid assessment. The doctor with psychosexual training is in a particularly good position to help such women reach a satisfactory conclusion and make sense of her situation. A student once asked this author if she found the work depressing. Interesting, exhausting challenging, frustrating possibly, but helping women with unplanned pregnancy is not depressing. There are perhaps very few situations where one can be of such benefit to the patient so quickly.

REFERENCES

Blair, M. (1983) Requests for termination of pregnancy, in *Practice of Psychosexual Medicine* (ed. K. Draper), John Libbey, London.

Christopher, E. (1989) Abortions in the 1980s. *British Journal of Family Planning*, **15**, 21-2.

Coles, R. (1983) Requests for abortion, in *Practice of Psychosexual Medicine* (ed. K. Draper), John Libbey, London.

Conway, M., Bolt, S., Cooper, E. *et al.* (1989) Long-term psychosexual problems after termination of pregnancy. *Institute of Psychosexual Medicine Newsletter*, **3**, 13-19.

Dagg, P. (1991) The psychological sequelae of therapeutic abortion – denied and completed. *American Journal of Psychiatry*, **148**, 578-85.

Fleissig, A. (1991) Unintended pregnancies and the use of contraception: changes from 1984 to 1989. *British Medical Journal*, **302**, 147.

Hutchinson, F. (1992) The Pill: a need for more information? *Novum*, **50**, 1-2.

Kaltreider, N.B., Goldsmith, S. and Margoles, A.J. (1979) The impact of mid-trimester abortion techniques on patient and staff. *American Journal of Obstetrics and Gynaecology*, **135**, 253–8.

OPCS Monitor (1991) *Legal Abortions 1990*, Office of Population Census and Surveys, London, July.

Potts, M., Diggory, P. and Peel, L. (1977) *Abortion*, Cambridge University Press, p. 3.

5

The wanted baby

Pauline Allen

SUMMARY

- Do I want a pregnancy?
- Infertility and the contraceptive consultation
- The couple
- The male factor

From their mutual penetration into the realms of supreme joy, the lovers bring back with them a spark of that light which we call life.
Marie Stopes (1926)

DO I WANT A BABY?

Marie Stopes wrote her book for lovers in the early days of contraception when ignorance of sexual matters abounded. Pregnancy was an inevitable consequence of married love, and contraception was used to space babies sensibly to allow the mothers to recuperate from childbirth. Today women can choose, with varied forms of contraception, either to have no babies at all, to have and space them, or to

defer them until the most favourable time. Among these many patterns
are women who fluctuate between wanting and not wanting babies.

Mrs N. married on the understanding that neither of them
wanted a baby. She was referred by a gynaecologist to
a specialist in psychosexual medicine because she was
still complaining of dyspareunia following a laparoscopy
and urethral dilatation, performed in an attempt to find
the cause for her pain. Nothing abnormal had been found.
She had been complaining of dyspareunia for 18 months
and there had been no intercourse for a year.

She was a smart business woman wearing a suit, who
came briskly into the room and sat down. She very quickly
began to tell the doctor how angry she was with the
people in the hospial. She had felt weak after the operation, so much so that she had to be off work for a whole
week. No one had warned her that it would be like this,
with so much abdominal pain and feeling so unwell and
her original problem had certainly not been resolved.

A simple question about the type of contraception she
was using brought an angry flood of tears and an out-
pouring of the story of how awful it was, and why she
was childless. Although she had married on the understanding that neither of them wanted to have children,
underneath she had been sure that if she changed her
mind it would be easy enough to persuade her husband
to think differently as well. As the years passed she
began to realize that she did want a baby but found she
was unable to sway her husband. She was angry that
he persisted in his rebellion against the family life that
she now desired; angry that he had been made redundant from his job; and angry that he should expect to
have sex with her when it was so painful.

Her immediate anger at the hospital staff was quickly reflected in the
speed with which she jumped at the subject of childlessness, almost as
if she was saying, 'Someone should have warned me that I would not be
able to change his mind about babies, even after 10 years of marriage.'

Because she was unable to share her ambivalent feelings about
motherhood with her husband, her fears of both having and being
without a baby were sublimated into a physical pain associated

with intercourse, so that their 'mutual penetration' became intolerable and inaccessible.

> She returned a few weeks later a much happier person. She said that the opportunity to share with the doctor her disappointment at the probability of not having a baby had enabled her to see things in a fresh light. It enabled her to talk about the grief that she felt for the baby she would not have, and she could see that it might be like a bereavement, full of different emotions, some anger some sadness, and even some relief that she would not have all the responsibilities that children bring. She loved her husband very much and wanted to spend her life with him. She had been able to talk about her disappointments with him and found that he had not deliberately been ignoring her needs, but that it had been too difficult for him to talk to her. They had made love several times without any pain.

Mrs. N. had learned that the problem did not lie in the fact that other people were ignoring the existence of her feelings, but that her ability to withhold and hide her feelings had been the cause of all her emotional and physical pain. She could now move on to the process of going through the various feelings of grief knowing that to make love involved a strong emotional as well as a physical element. Now she had brought her ambivalent feelings about a baby into the open with her husband it had become an easier sharing process, and there was less pain. She was still undecided about whether she wanted a baby but the dilemma was no longer expressed as a physical problem.

INFERTILITY AND THE CONTRACEPTIVE CONSULTATION

During the contraceptive consultation it is difficult to remember that some of the women or couples will be consulting their doctor at a later date because of an infertility problem. Society is geared to the assumption that Marie Stopes made all those years ago, that every couple will bring forth a child when they want one; in other words, our society is constructed for the fertile.

Money is channelled into family planning and abortion services, and the maternity and child health services, but little is spent on the infertile. Such an arrangement adds to the suspicions of subfertile couples that their needs are not being listened to.

It is actually not an insignificant problem when it is remembered that for one in six couples, at some time in their lives, the wanted baby will not materialize without some medical intervention. These couples include those trying for their first baby as well as those who are having trouble conceiving their second or subsequent baby. Such couples suffer constant emotional pain, and can feel very isolated in society for, like all of us, their expectations of becoming normal adults and parents had been taken for granted, and it is only when a pregnancy does not ensue that they begin to realize that they may not be 'normal'.

The desperate and bitter isolation is often made worse when friends become pregnant, or inquiring relatives make comments such as, 'Isn't it time you started thinking about settling down with a family?' The emotional pain is usually hidden from friends and relatives, but may be shared within the anonymity of an infertility clinic, together with the physical pains such as dyspareunia, and the sexual problems of nonconsummation, non-ejaculation and impotence which may accompany the problem of infertility.

In the contraceptive clinic plans and expectations about a family can be shared with the doctor very early when discussing contraception. A simple question like, 'I wonder if you are considering a family at any stage?', before writing out the repeat Pill prescription may well introduce another dimension to the routine demands of contraception, especially if the woman has been on the Pill for many years or is well into her 30s. The answer may be like any other answer, very vague – this year, next year, sometime, never – but it not only gives the doctor an opportunity of discussing possible problems that could arise, for both her and her partner if a pregnancy is not attempted until the woman is much older, but also may give some indication of her feelings about babies.

Contraception is often considered to be just about stopping babies, but it also says a great deal about having a good sex life without the fear of a pregnancy. Why are doctors so afraid to bring up the topic of sex with their patients when discussing contraception? It is so important to elicit possible problems early on. Is she wanting a good sex life with no babies? Is she wanting to delay her family until the 'right time', and also have a good sex life? Is she wanting to enjoy an active sex life with her partner without the obvious responsibilities that a baby will produce, at the present time or maybe forever? Is she having a sex life at all – or is it just that everyone else takes the Pill when they are in a stable relationship, engaged or getting married? The assumption that sexual intercourse has taken place when the woman has been on the Pill for many years is common, but it is not always justified, and appropriate comments or questions to clarify the situation should be mandatory.

Mrs H. had hidden the nonconsummation of their marriage for eight years. She had requested repeat prescriptions for the Pill, avoided examinations by having a period or a pressing engagement, and had also moved house and general practitioner (GP) on several occasions. Eventually she plucked up courage to approach her new female doctor, saying that she wanted to have a baby and thought it sensible to have a smear before stopping the Pill. She did not mention the lack of intercourse.

The doctor noticed the hesitancy in her preparation to get on to the couch and remove her underwear for the examination. She looked like a young girl, despite her 28 years, rather like a china doll with neatly parted and waved hair, no make-up and wearing a summer dress with puffed sleeves. She sat up on the couch with her arms clutching her knees and to the doctor's comment about her apparent reluctance to be examined she began to talk about the lack of penetration in their sex life. Nobody had asked her about sex before and if they had the answer would have been 'it is all right', for they did enjoy a degree of intimacy when she achieved an orgasm with manual stimulation. It was only now that they wanted a baby that the situation had become a problem.

She said, 'We waited all these years deliberately until the time was right.' Their world was now ready for a baby; they both had good jobs, their new house was completely furnished, and most of their friends were now having babies. It was just this physical block and the shape of her vagina that was causing the difficulty.

They had tried on so many occasions but her husband's penis just would not go in.

The doctor was able to do a smear quite easily, probably because there had been some introital stretching with their attempts at intercourse, and she tried to reassure her that there did not appear to be a physical block in her vagina. However, she felt that more time was needed to explore this woman's difficulties, and she referred her to a special psychosexual clinic.

Nowadays, with a national cervical screening programme in place, someone like Mrs H. may not manage to avoid a smear for so long, but she would certainly have managed to find some effective way of keeping both doctors and her husband away from her emotional fears surrounding intercourse until she wanted a baby: if not away from the actual physical examination, as had happened here. The patient has to want some changes to be made before treatment can begin to be effective, but Mrs H. could not acknowledge her own desire to have intercourse and all that it might mean for her. However, now it was for a baby she felt that it was a suitably acceptable reason to approach her doctor about such an uncomfortable topic.

It took Mr and Mrs H. almost a year to achieve intercourse and there followed 18 months of infertility before the psychosexual doctor met them again, this time in the infertility clinic. Mrs H. had changed into a confident woman compared with the little girl that had appeared originally. A simple ovulation induction regime proved successful and they now have a healthy young son.

To those who decide the time is right for the wanted baby, a pregnancy is achieved by the majority of couples within the first two years of trying to conceive. Modern contraception has encouraged people to feel in control of their lives so that when its use is discontinued, expectations of an ensuing pregnancy occurring immediately are very high. When one does not occur, the emotional anxieties begin to feature very largely in the daily agenda of the woman, and sometimes of the couple.

The most common single problem, accounting for a quarter of all infertility problems, is that of sperm defect or dysfunction. Nearly a half are caused by a mixture of female problems, another quarter by unexplained reasons, and finally 6% due to coital problems. These are useful figures to remember when trying to put infertility problems into perspective and form a balanced view of the cause, if any. However, they do not give any indication of the amount of emotional disturbance felt by the individuals involved. The feelings of failure, utter disbelief and sometimes denial that they are in this situation can be seen in such statements as, 'We're not ready for children yet' or 'We're quite busy enough with our dogs at the moment'.

THE COUPLE

Often a woman has managed to be seen on her own during many visits to her GP and the gynaecology outpatient clinic without the inclusion of her partner. He may well have attended the clinics but somehow, because he was not invited into the consultations, he remained in the waiting room, on the fringe of this 'women's world'. How does this happen? Patients' understanding of infertility problems revolve around the premise that it is almost entirely a female deficiency. Just in the same way that society has equipped itself for the fertile, so all assumptions and efforts at treatment have been tailored to the female side of the problem. Therefore it is so often the woman who appears first in the surgery with the statement, 'We've been trying for a baby for so many months now, and I just don't seem to be able to get pregnant.' Because it is the woman who is there in front of the doctor it is usually she who is the focus of all the initial tests, without any discussion between the couple and the doctor. Such discussion with the couple, to exclude any psycho-sexual problems, is as important as the gamut of blood tests that are carried out. It can also act as a baseline for the recognition of developing difficulties during sometimes lengthy treatment.

Although it had been suspected for some time that male causes for infertility existed, it is only comparatively recently that problems related to sperm and their function have been shown to be the largest single cause. It will take many years for the varied cultures throughout the world to inwardly digest this particular truth. Doctors can make small inroads into the unjustified belief that it is always the woman's fault, by seeing couples together from the beginning of treatment and not just patting the man on the back and saying, 'That's a fine sperm count, old chap, no problem there.' A change in approach will make it less likely that the woman will be left with all the anxieties and doubts placed on her own ability to produce this wanted baby. In any event, it is possible that there may be cause for the problem in both partners.

At the present, specialized infertility clinics exist where couples are invited to attend together for their appointments. The joint interviews can provide an extra dimension in the realm of differential diagnosis if the interactions between the couple are noted. Often it will be the first time that these two individuals have been seen together. There are many scenarios that give insight into the two separate sides of the relationship, and the difficulties within it, that might well go unnoticed or ignored in the traditional medical models of treatment.

Mr and Mrs B. attended their first appointment anxiously together, but Mr B. had to keep retiring to the car park during the hour-long discussion because he felt faint in hospitals. Mrs B. apologised profusely for him and protected him from any further appointments. Many months later during treatment when she was obviously putting on a brave face at the appearance of yet another period, a comment about her fierce ability to protect not only her husband from his fears of hospitals, but also him and the doctors from her devastation and grief at the feared inevitable childlessness, enabled her to pour out, with tears and words, all her anger at the situation. The clinic counsellor was then able to visit them at home and have an open discussion with them both. They hope to resume further infertility treatment after a few months of reflection.

In this case the observation and interpretation of the wife's need to protect her husband and others helped in the management of the infertile situation that the couple found themselves in.

Mrs F. marched into the clinic well ahead of her husband. She immediately launched into the story of how she was the most interesting case of polycystic ovaries that her GP had seen in years. Eventually the doctor managed to bring Mr F. into the discussion and made a comment about how important it was to hear both sides of the story. A short while later he felt able to reveal, for the first time ever to anyone, that he had undescended testes. He had read about it, and knew what the probable outcome would be, and now he wanted to be examined without his wife present. The anger that she felt was overwhelming, too much for the doctor to do other than acknowledge. Whether it was due to the sudden realization of ensuing childlessness with this man, fury at the secret he had kept or the fact that he was now the one with the interesting medical condition, the doctor was not sure. What was certain was that she had kept him out of the consultation, ignoring him in the room, and in the same way had kept him out of all investigations by the normally very efficient GP. After several more visits they decided not to return.

Noticing the way in which couples interact together in the clinic or surgery can give an insight into how they interact together at home, and so play an important part in the help that can be offered to them. This type of counselling can be carried out by experienced clinicians at the same time as discussions about the advantages and disadvantages of investigations and treatments. Couples need the opportunity to weigh up their chances of a pregnancy so that they can make an informed choice about the direction to take. Sometimes this involves the painful realization of lost hopes and dreams.

On occasions the two individuals appear to have coalesced into one, in such a way that the wanted baby has become an amalgamation of their mutual desires. Their own individual personalities appear to have been lost many months or even years before. Although they must both have their own emotions and feelings about being childless, it can be very difficult for these to be respected by each other, let alone the doctor.

Mr and Mrs E., a wealthy Indian couple, had been trying to achieve a pregnancy since their arranged marriage two years previously. Mrs E. was frightened and withdrawn at her first visit to the infertility clinic at the hospital, but seemed to be somewhat relieved to find a female doctor present. Mr E. gave the history and spoke for her. They adhered to all the investigations and treatment regimes with precision. She was diagnosed as having polycystic ovarian disease, and underwent a year of gonadotrophin therapy to induce cycles of ovulation, but she still did not become pregnant. Only on one occasion did the doctor manage to examine Mrs E. on her own. She hinted at her despair about her failure to conceive, and at the lack of fun with sex, but her allegiance to her upbringing and to her husband prevented her from letting go of any of her own feelings.

Several times on visits to the hospital, tears would appear but they would be stifled by her husband's words, 'Don't worry, she will be all right soon.' They were both sad when it was agreed that treatment should stop, but the doctor was again told not to worry as they would be fine. The only treatment left to them was to consider *in vitro* fertilization, where the fertilizing power of the sperm could be studied as well as ovulation. This idea must have posed difficulties for Mr E. but he could not share them with any member of the clinic staff.

Several months elapsed before Mr E. telephoned to say that they would like a private referral to be admitted on to the assisted conception programme at a nearby centre: he asked for it to be done immediately because he had got his wife in the mood for it now. An offer to come and discuss it again was firmly but politely refused.

The decisions of this couple regarding a pregnancy and the chosen method towards success had been made outside the medical setting. They made their own choices, showing that doctors can provide every type of counselling for couples, but they will only be able to use what is comfortable for them. Counselling is a two-way process and no-one can be forced into sharing their anxieties.

THE SECOND BABY

Many couples who have had problems conceiving their first baby have found no trouble in becoming pregnant for a second or subsequent time. But what about the agony of those whose second baby does not materialize? The women themselves often say, 'I suppose I shouldn't be making such a fuss because I am so lucky to have one baby.' For those setting up infertility self-help groups, one of the first questions always seems to be, 'Do we have separate groups for those with and without children?' Couples with trouble conceiving a second child are certainly not recognized in the statistic which says that only 4% of women remain involuntarily childless at the menopause, but fortunately they have been included in Hull's figures of one in six couples seeking help for infertility at some stage in their lives (Hull, Glazener, Kelly *et al.*, 1985).

The reliance on the efficacy of birth control is so great that a woman's expectation of control over her own reproductive capacity is equally high. When contraception, pregnancy and contraception again have followed in an easy sequence, the non-occurrence of the expected pregnancy comes as a great shock.

The gradual progression of one of the most common female disorders, that of polycystic ovarian disease, with the occurrence of oligomenorrhoea and in some case hirsutes and weight gain compounds the whole problem. The resultant despondency can lead on to excessive eating, an altered body image and the attempted killing of all sexual attractiveness in revenge for her body not performing to the reproductive expectations built up over many years. It is possible to help some of these women to gain insight into how their anger is being directed at their immediate family as well as themselves.

With time to reflect on their own needs, as well as that of the family, one finds that there can be as much ambivalence about the desire for a second child as for the first baby, again particularly in those women who had no problems conceiving the first time. Couples do not appear in surgeries or clinics until the first child is about to start school at four or five years old. It is as though there is a sudden panic at the realization that their first child has nearly left home and maybe they have left it too late. It can be seen here how bereavement becomes one of the emotions felt by a woman in this situation, often leading to mounting tension within the relationship.

Mrs S. was desperate for a second child when she first arrived at the clinic. Her first child was conceived easily and was now about to start school. She had developed polycystic ovarian disease and was grossly overweight. A regime of ovulation induction was carried out successfully for six months but no pregnancy was achieved. The doctor was wondering how she could manage the next visit because she knew that Mrs S. could not afford an assisted conception programme. She need not have worried. Mrs S. hurried into the clinic saying that she had made up her own mind. 'I've finished grieving for the baby that has not happened,' she said. 'I want to live my own life for a while. I'm starting a job next week.' She had been through a lot of heartache, seeing friends and relatives with babies, but she had managed to lose some weight and with the help of the clinic staff she had been able to make her own choices.

Mrs S. had continuous support throughout her treatment in an environment where she had been encouraged to make her own decisions, including whether or not to have treatment, and when to stop. Others need more than this, especially when there is the added problem of mental or physical disability in the first baby. It is not just the obvious problem of managing to cope with another child at home, but consideration of whether there is a likelihood of the next baby having the same problem. Genetic advice must be sought, and discussions with a counsellor and perhaps self-help groups should be offered. Much of the personal assessment for the two individuals concerned is to do with how much fault they attribute to themselves for the disability in the child.

Mrs P. was seen initially in a psychosexual clinic following the birth of her first child who suffered from osteogenesis imperfecta (brittle bone disease). Intercourse was extremely painful. She was unable to gain any insight into how angry she was with the doctors for not diagnosing the problem correctly so that some fractures occurred during the baby's delivery, but she was also angry with her husband for possibly causing some fractures when he lay on her having intercourse.

The previous fun of lovemaking had led to a wanted pregnancy, but it had caused so much pain now for her and her baby. How could she possibly enjoy it again? She did not want any more children and therefore there was no need for intercourse. She decided not to attend for further help with the psychosexual problem because of lack of progress.

Three years later she appeared at the infertility clinic having decided herself, a year before, that the time was

right for another baby. She looked surprised when the
doctor asked if she was enjoying lovemaking again, as
though that painful time had not existed.

The power of time to heal both pain and anger can sometimes be
surprising, and doctors have to accept that they will often never know
if the work they have done with a patient has played any part in the
healing process.

THE MALE FACTOR

As already stated, a quarter of all infertility problems are due to sperm
defect or dysfunction. The male factor also plays a part in the 6%
of couples with coital problems. However, this latter figure does not
include the secondary coital problems that arise as a result of investigations or treatments for the infertility.

Thexton (1992) writes about 'reluctant fathers', where the
men openly express their dislike of fatherhood. Such men are
not seen in infertility clinics, but the ones who do come are those
who have covert, often unconscious feelings that lead to difficulty with ejaculation or impotence. Such problems may develop
when there is some change in their lives which leads to the possibility of pending fatherhood. Nonconsummation is often a mixture
of fears in both partners relating to damage to one or other of
them.

Some infertility tests such as the postcoital test, or the need to
have intercourse on specific days, can result in varying degrees of
impotence. Longer lasting episodes have been seen to occur following the discovery of azoospermia. Ambivalence about the wish for
a baby, which has already been described in women and in couples,
may lie at a deep level in the man. Contraceptive decisions are
frequently affected by such mixed feelings, but changes in contraception can also expose previously unsuspected and hidden
ambivalence.

Miss A. and Mr T., both professional business people,
had lived together for 13 years with no intention of
having any children. Miss A. had suddenly decided in
her mid-30s that she wanted a baby and had stopped
taking her Pill. Mr T. could no longer ejaculate, and

from having a very satisfying and full sex life, they had resorted to intercourse at midcycle only, using masturbation and injection of semen with a syringe, as had been suggested by a sex therapist.

At the infertility clinic they expressed their desire to proceed quickly with achieving a baby because as Mr T. said, 'We are getting quite old for babies, but we have the rest of our lives to deal with the sex problem.' He did not want to be seen separately for his problem.

The doctor decided to press on quickly with an examination of Miss A. She seemed to be the most anxious and to be doing most of the talking. Sex really was not much fun now since the problem started and she had not had an orgasm either. She felt that she had put pressure on him in the first place about not having children and it seemed so sad, now that they both wanted a baby, that it had to be conceived in such a cold manner. The suggestion that she could relieve some of the pressure and enjoy sex again if she wanted to seemed a revelation to her.

It was a brief encounter but things improved dramatically over the next few weeks while investigations were taking place. They were able to make love whenever they chose, and he usually ejaculated, only having occasional difficulty around the time of ovulation. In fact, she became pregnant within a couple of months and said she was sure it was one of the natural times. Mr T. did not want, or need, treatment or outside help with his problem. He had been able to ejaculate again within the security of their relationship when Miss A. was able to share her knowledge and understanding of the pressures she had been imposing on him.

The existence of absolute sterility is rare and therefore the door of hope is left open for the majority of couples. Such hope can at times become unbearable: 'If only someone would say there was no hope, we could begin to adjust.' Perhaps doctors need to help these, and others, to look at their fears of the closed door so that it can be included more often in their range of choices.

The wanted baby

Tell us of pain. And the prophet said:
Your pain is the breaking of the shell that encloses your
understanding.
Even as the stone of the fruit must break, that its heart
may stand in the sun, so must you know pain.
And could you keep your heart in wonder at the daily
miracles of your life, your pain would not seem less
wondrous than your joy;
And you would accept the seasons of your heart, even as
you have always accepted the seasons that pass over your
fields.
And you would watch with serenity through the winters of
your grief.

Kahlil Gibran (1926)

REFERENCES

Gibran, K. (1926) *The Prophet*, William Heinemann, London.
Hull, M.G.R., Glazener, C.M.A., Kelly, N.J. *et al.* (1985) Population study
of causes, treatment and outcome of infertility. *British Medical Journal*,
291, 1693–7.
Stopes, M. (1926) Married Love 18 edn G.P. Putnam Sons, London.
Thexton, R. (1992) Ejaculatory difficulties, in *Psychosexual Medicine* (ed.
R. Lincoln), Chapman & Hall, London.

6

The man and the method

Andrew Stainer-Smith

SUMMARY

- The stereotypes
  'Man the hunter'
  'Men hate condoms'
  'Contraception is left to the woman'
  'Men need to be in control'
  'Men are aggressive'
- Psychosexual skills

INTRODUCTION

Why do men consult doctors so little about contraception? One may assume that they do not have strong feelings on the subject, or what feelings they have are aired and dealt with outside a doctor's surgery. A less satisfactory but more likely explanation is that men are conditioned by their upbringing to believe that they should have adequate internal resources to deal with any conflicts that arise. Is this the case? Few contraceptive textbooks deal with men's feelings, and they offer little more than chapters on the mechanics of condom use and vasectomy. Where attitudes are mentioned, they tend to come over as generalizations or personal assumptions of the writer. This chapter has been written after listening to the views of many actual men.

To find a current cross-section of men's ideas about contraception, this author interviewed about 20 men in some depth over three months, giving them opportunities to air their feelings. Often their initial responses to probings were in the form of neat, acceptable replies, but as they relaxed their attitude changed to become more questioning, and at times there was considerable distress. Men were seen at home, alone, and in comfortable surroundings. This author has known them all for some time in the capacity of either their GP or their family's GP. Men were selected who differed widely, ranging from one who was proud of his title as 'the virgin cracker', through to married and ummarried couples, the sample including two men of over 50 years.

The overwhelming attitude of men to this approach was that they wanted to ask whether their feelings were normal. They had clear preconceptions of ordinary male behaviour against which they considered their own feelings, identifying areas where they felt different. This sense of difference had over the years given rise to varying degrees of anxiety, and several of the men appeared to value the opportunity to talk in more depth.

In the present chapter this study has been used, as well as the glimpses of men's attitudes to contraception seen during many years in general practice. Because of the strength of the stereotypes some of these common assumptions about male behaviour have been used as headings under which to consider the varied feelings of different individuals.

THE STEREOTYPES

'Man the hunter'

The active, predatory young and older men who described the hunting phase of their lives in detail, were at pains to explain how they were different. They pointed out that they were just as much approached by women as making the first moves themselves.

It is well known that enquiring about those things that an individual dislikes in others may uncover feelings about the parts of himself with which he is uncomfortable: what has been described as his hidden shadow (Samuels, 1985). A man may imply, 'Others behave like this all the time, but I am different.' In the next breath he is likely to explain that all men have an instinct to prey on women.

Does contraception come into this at all? This author believes it does, for contraception may be seen as a defence from being preyed upon (trapped in pregnancy). It can also be a protection against sexually transmitted disease, and it can be a useful barrier for those men who do not want too much emotional closeness with a woman.

> Mr. A. had been a stud and was proud of it. He had moved down from London and spent some time teaching the locals a few lessons. Now after settling into married life he is running a garage and car hire business and is well known in the local community for giving a helping hand. In the past girls had fallen into three categories; some who were seen as fair game; some who would be avoided; and some who were in need of his protection. He was asked how he used to decide about contraception? 'Often you cannot decide if you are carried away.' The doctor asked, 'Did you treat them all the same? You seem a gentle chap to me.' After a pause he flushed. 'It was the quiet ones I worried about – sometimes. The ones you could hurt. I always used condoms with them, because in a way you felt they shouldn't be doing it. If you had met them somewhere else they were the ones you could marry.'

So although young men out hunting may at times not carry contraception, when they do it may be to protect themselves against physical and perhaps emotional dangers, or occasionally to protect their quarry.

'Contraception is left to the woman'

Men are unlikely to admit that they consider contraception to be the woman's business but again the shadow is there. 'A lot of other men do,' they say. Perhaps it is because many men are nervous about their sexuality. They stir quickly and not always when expected, and they are not used to the idea of saying 'No' and waiting for a more suitable time. On the assumption he wants sex, he may be carrying condoms. On the other hand, he hopes that any girl who lets him get carried away will have thought about it in advance and also have protection.

> Mr B., now in his early 40s, used to have a wild time in the evenings after his rock concerts. Now he is a vigorous homemaker/house parent and his wife is the main wage earner. 'I did not really like the nympho-maniacs, and after a bit I got to saying no.' 'Why?' 'It seemed that they all wanted babies, underneath. And even if you were using condoms they were pretending, and hoping to themselves that it was for real. They were lonely really. I did not want kids, but even without that risk they were behaving like babies themselves. Within a few days you couldn't shake them off.' 'And you didn't want to have to cope with that?' the doctor asked, paus-ing before he continued. 'Children are very important to you now.' Mr. B. thought and replied, 'I wish I could have them myself.' As the doctor left, Mr. B. said, 'We have been talking about another child, but perhaps it is too late now.'

Mr. B.'s present lifestyle shows him comfortable with his feminine side. He does not have to be 'macho', to prove his masculinity, but now regrets he has taken so long to want children for himself. In his youth his fear of being trapped made him extremely nervous about leaving contraception to the other party, but also somewhat guilty about his behaviour, with a degree of insight into the problems of his victims.

'Men hate condoms'

There is no doubt that dislike for the condom is common. The clearest description met was, 'Once you have gone bareback, there is nothing like it!' Men dislike having to pause, and may find losing their erection at this stage a problem, even after years of use.

On the other hand some men can be very fond of condoms. They are old friends and remind us of exciting times. One man told me their loving was dull until one family camping holiday when she asked him to get some to save messing their sleeping bag. Now when they can at last afford hotels they still take condoms with them on holiday to add a spice of excitement.

Conversely, as a means of slowing down excitement the use of the sheath is not always helpful.

> Mr. C. has severe premature ejaculation and he put it this way. 'Imagine what it is like. You put on a condom to stop coming. Sometimes I come when she is watching me put it on, and if I get inside I am likely to go soft and it will come off before I ejaculate.'
>
> He was desperately in love with and excited by his younger wife. He had coped by not lying close to her in bed, and when they came to make love he tried with condoms to show willing, but it did not help. His problem led to such stress that his wife had an affair with someone else and got pregnant. By this time he was completely impotent. Later, when his jealousy was out in the open, his anger exploded one day as she went out to playgroup in clothes revealing most of her body. He was able to express his need to have more of her for himself, and when she withdrew her exposure to the privacy of their bedroom, he became potent again.

Interrupting sex to put on a condom is a problem, and not only for the young. Some older men enjoy prolonged lovemaking during which their erection comes and goes. Deciding when to put it on is stressful. It is difficult getting them on the right way round in the dark. Some flavoured or fun varieties are not lubricated and are difficult to apply. One youngster said, 'Girls are not like blokes. You find you have just got her ready when . . . bother it. Half a minute to 'get dressed' and she's gone off.'

Men do not like buying them. They talk of the embarrassment of feeling that shop assistants believe condoms are for a mistress rather than a regular partner. They do not trust mail order companies not to divulge details to other sales agencies. Bulk buys are perceived as being generic and possibly substandard. A more popular method than over-the-counter sales is by using a credit card to buy from an advertisement in a woman's magazine. Selling here is seen as conferring some special degree of approval – and can be left more easily for the partner to do. At the other extreme, one young man told me, 'It is best to make a joke of it. Go up to a young assistant in a chemist with a packet and ask her what this sort are like.' Not necessarily a joke for the shop assistant. If this man, with his general

lack of embarrassment, finds buying a problem, then it must deter
some men altogether.

Not all complaints about condoms should be taken at face value.

> Mr D. complained that using a condom often left him
> soft with no erection and his wife was disappointed. He
> was married with two children and the doctor felt
> surprised by the complaint. Later he told how he had
> recently led a discussion about contraception at his
> church youth club. It was OK to talk at church, but at
> home it was difficult. 'Women don't understand how
> men find it difficult to talk.' He added, 'Whenever she
> talks to me about condoms, it turns me off, and I
> wouldn't want her to try and put one on me.' This
> sounded like a polite complaint and the doctor listened
> quietly. Mr. D. went on, 'If I join in the conversation when
> she goes on about coming off the Pill, she seems to get
> excited and silly and I don't like that.' It was becoming
> clear that his real worry was that his wife might want
> another baby. The doctor realized that these two people
> were not communicating. He observed the house – a few
> essential jobs done, but in need of partial rebuilding. He
> knew that Mr. D. was a carpenter who did his own small
> building jobs on the side. Why was his own home so
> neglected? The doctor reflected, 'Sarah has to wait a long
> time to get what she wants from you.' Mr. D. laughed
> uncomfortably and other subjects were talked about.
> That was a while ago. Sarah is now off the Pill, much
> happier and they are using condoms. He is on the waiting
> list for a vasectomy, and as he says, 'It's time I did my bit.'

Here was a man who was complaining that condoms made him soft,
but discussion with his doctor allowed him to talk more freely with
his wife and to identify his real worries that his wife might want more
children. However, when they could communicate openly he discovered his fears were groundless and they could use condoms happily
again.

'Men need to be in control'

Control is an important theme in psychosexual medicine. The

matter of who is in control colours many psychosexual problems. Impotence may be a dumb protest against a controlling partner. Desire for sex can evaporate when advances are rebuffed, or one partner demands attention in circumstances that they know are unevenly disempowering. Vaginismus enters self-perpetuating cycles when the woman is kept from being allowed to take charge of herself. Premature ejaculation is frequently a feature of a man frightened of what could happen if his feelings were truly out of control.

Likewise it is useful to look at how contraceptive decisions are made and where the power base lies in the compromise. Many men were keen to explain how their decision had been made jointly with their partner. However, when given the opportunity to talk further it often became clear that one partner had relinquished more control than the other.

In the following sections some of the conscious and unconscious feelings about the common methods are dicussed.

Condom use

Condom use is traditionally the man's decision. It is seen as good manners, caring and safe. It protects both parties, but particularly the woman from something noxious. The guidelines seem clear for the promiscuous and those in stable partnerships, but these are artificial distinctions. A man may not want to use a condom for what it implies. He may have had very few partners and not perceive himself as any threat. He may be keen to show how he respects his girlfriend and not want to view her as source of disease. In those circumstances he may well step away from condoms for what they imply and risk coitus interruptus or nothing. As she says, 'I don't want the sort of man who needs condoms.'

The cap

The cap lies in the vagina. It is a temporarily accommodated guest without eyes or ears. Provided it does its job, it is tolerated, and guests are fine to have around if you feel well. If you are not feeling so well, they are not so fine.

Most doctors are familiar with the issues that a cap brings to the fore for a woman, but the feelings it arouses in the man are less well studied. Men have been heard to use combative phrases to describe it. 'I don't fancy catching my weapon on that', and 'What if I knock it into the wrong position?' For them it is not an unnoticed companion in their private place.

> Mr E. is now separated from his wife. Things had been strained for some time. She had asked him to go back to condoms 'because of the mess'. Later she announced, 'You can leave them off if you want now.' Mr E. said he could cope with the cap, but could not understand how hurt he felt when she told him she had been using it for several weeks before she told him. 'I had hoped it meant we were getting closer', he said, 'but that thing [the cap] was worse because I couldn't see it.'

Intrauterine contraceptive devices (IUCDs)

An IUCD invests much control in the doctor. Maybe it has been discussed, perhaps even with both parties. All the same, it is a foreign body. It is hard, metallic, and considered an abortifacient by some people, as well as being seen as a possible source of disease. Men can frequently feel threads and worry about dislodging it. One man said, 'I knew when she had a coil in because I could taste the metal when I kissed her.' There is often disbelief that something so tiny can work. When a small sample of men were asked to rank contraceptive methods in order of efficiency, all men put IUCDs bottom of the list.

Some of the anxiety about the method may reflect the general awareness of the safety of modern contraceptive pills and the threat of pelvic infection, even although that is a small risk in multipara who are in a stable relationship. Many people are well informed and may wish to discuss the risks of specific infections such as chlamydia. Despite reassurance one can hear a certain 'I told you so' attitude from men towards the coil if complications arise. This can be interpreted as being an expression of healthy caution about a contraceptive method that asks for such a degree of trust in the doctor from the woman and her partner.

Medicine, and in particular contraception, is an intrusive business. In contraceptive work doctors frequently pick up echoes of dissatisfaction with a bad experience in the past. Either partner may have been to a genitourinary clinic, which can heighten their fear of infection, and often adds an extra sense of guilt to those who are not completely happy with their sexuality. Women may have had an unexpected instrumental delivery. These experiences leave scars, sometimes of an unexpected kind.

> Mr F. is a hard-working electrician who often worked late. He said, 'I wouldn't like her to have a coil, she'd find it too embarrassing.' He is a man who keeps an awkward distance from medical events when he is wanted. When his wife has migraine, or grandmother's blood specimen needs taking to the laboratory, he is always too far away to help. Later he told me about his wife's delivery. She needed stitches and he hoped to get out of the delivery room, but somehow he ended up holding the baby. The midwife and his wife said what a pair they made in the low chair across the room, but all he was thinking of was the doctor's hand inside his wife, particularly as at the same time she was smiling. 'No, no-one is going to give her a coil, thank you.'

Most men have heard of expulsion and perforation. A woman came asking for a second IUCD 10 years and a second marriage after being perforated by her first device. The doctor was amazed after this failure, although in some ways it was a sensible request. She was now hypertensive, so the Pill was not suitable, and as she was no longer nulliparous, the risk of another perforation was slight. But the doctor wanted to hear the reasons why she was prepared to try something again when it had caused problems the first time.

The first coil had been resented. The marriage had already gone wrong and she seemed to blame her first husband more than the doctor for the perforation. 'In a way I was glad it had to be removed [even by laparoscopy]. From then on we used condoms, but not very often.' He was a policeman with no sense of fun. 'At least it kept his truncheon covered.' Now she wanted all barriers removed so as to welcome her new man, and he was worth some risk.

The Pill

Who controls the Pill? There is no doubt that it is in the woman's hands, but men appear to have just as many worries about the health risks as women. However, these worries are often not expressed very loudly, but may be heard as asides: 'How can you tell if she is

taking it?' Or reported by their partners: 'Those clever doctors may
let you down again.' 'They don't tell you about all the side-effects.'
'Have you ever read the pack insert?' There is rarely an opportunity
to answer such questions adequately and they ask for a considerable
degree of trust from the man. A psychosexual doctor may be
prompted to ask why he feels he has to answer questions. Are they
really questions or a request that the man should not be asked to put
so much trust in something unnatural and a drug? One caring
husband said, 'I wish I could take it instead of her.' Again, asking
men to rank effectiveness, the Pill came below condoms in their
perception.

A young man said, 'When they are on the Pill, it is as if they are
pregnant. They put on weight and it makes them want babies. I would
always use a condom too.' Again, the feeling of the Pill being a risk
was put in this way: 'A girl on the Pill may change her mind and
stop it; perhaps after making love, especially if it was good.'

And what does the Pill control? Certainly if taken correctly it does
provide excellent fertility control. But at a deeper level, the Pill
interferes with natural cycles. Does it matter that a couple loses touch
with the moon and tides? No-one directly complained of this, but
in many discussions there surfaced an agreement that nature was being
interfered with. One man asked, 'If she got pregnant on the Pill, would
the child's periods be affected later?' As the child is mother to the
adult, we want the child to have a natural, healthy start.

In talk of hormones, people mentioned steroids, hair growth,
infertility, osteoporosis, cystic ovaries, baldness, libido changes and
homosexuality. The word 'hormone' has become tainted because of
its association with steroids and drugs. Men are cautious about what
may be going on when their partner is on the Pill. Some felt that
premenstrual tension was worse on the Pill, 'even though she gets
some break'. The tension was seen as a build up from the drugs over
the 21 days of Pill taking.

The rhythm method

The rhythm method implies a great deal of control but is poorly
understood by many men. Several of those spoken to thought the
rhythm method meant withdrawal. Once clarified, it was clear that
there were many misunderstandings. The days after menstruation were
regarded as safer than those before. However, those couples who

did use it seemed to share their understandings and were happy. As expected, these were couples with a keen desire for the natural, or strong religious beliefs. They were aware of confusing medical advice on timings, and had their own feelings about what was safe despite the advice. Usually both the man and the woman knew when she ovulated, and this closeness was apparent in discussion. 'It puts a brake on us', said one man. 'If we have been cross with each other, she doesn't always ovulate, and then we have to wait.'

Withdrawal

Can withdrawal be considered the ultimate test of control for the man? It involves fully potent sex up to a point that only he can recognize. Most men have tried it at some time, and talked excitedly about the experience until it came to describing the difficult bit. In addition to recognizing the importance of his own control, several said it was impossible if, at the last moment, the woman grabbed hold with her arms or legs and held him in. These men were describing risky sex, and the group must contain a number whose enjoyment is particularly connected with the risk of conception.

Vasectomy

Loss of fertility might be considered the moment when the man becomes unarmed. 'Have a vasectomy and join the club.' It is impossible not to have attitudes to vasectomy, though the overwhelming first response to the event was that it was 'a small job and made no difference'.

There is evidence that the quality of marriage for the woman may improve after vasectomy (Adler, Cook, Gray *et al.*, 1981). On the other hand, there is a measurable regret for some men which leads to requests for reversal (Howard, 1982).

Mr G. is a fireman and one of those men who described his vasectomy as a 'small job'. He then reassured himself by saying it was a difficult part of life at last put behind them and that they could relax. Sex was the same and the family complete. The doctor felt a strong hint that discussion of the matter should now be completed, and it was for the time being. Later Mr G. relaxed and was able to say how much more time he had at home, particularly because 'we don't seem to need so much sex now, and anyway the children need so much of our time'. Some time later the discussion returned to contraception. 'Did it take long to decide about a vasectomy?' 'No. She said . . . . , well, we agreed that I would do my bit, and it didn't matter who was done.' There was a long silence. 'I wonder if your wife would have decided so quickly about being sterilized herself?' After a pause he replied, 'You know, in a way, I thought more about it afterwards. It took me several months to get used to it. At first I thought I was bound to go off sex, but it is no good getting cross about it.' Mr G. became visibly upset, and it was necessary to arrange a follow-up consultation later, which had a satisfactory outcome.

It is suggested that sterilization requires grieving. All sterilization involves a loss – a loss of fertility. Though it may be by vasectomy or tubal ligation or naturally, as at the menopause, it is not necessarily welcomed. Mr G. was left numb and empty after the procedure. It was not acceptable for him to be angry with his wife for pushing him to do it. Although there was some camaraderie and group support in 'joining the club', he needed help to see why he went off sex and is only now enjoying it again two years later.

What features of the grief reaction should be expected. Emptiness, denial, anger and later readjustment to a world that will never be the same. This is not a time to hand over control on the spur of the moment. Doctors are sometimes asked by a partner to arrange vasectomy for the spouse. It is essential to determine how the request has come about; perhaps interviewing the man alone. Doctors may be asked for advice when a choice for a vasectomy or tubal ligation seems even handed. An important parameter to consider is to identify who would grieve least from losing their fertility.

Mr H. came requesting vasectomy. He was a small businessman whose wife helped in the playgroup. Their children were older and starting secondary school. The doctor pictured his wife as an intensely earthbound mother putting continued efforts into child rearing and understanding the needs of parents and their desire to procreate. Mr H. spent most of his time at the shop.

The doctor asked him how he would feel about never being able to father a child again. He paused, quietened and said how he loathed the shop. He had hoped that his wife would put more hours in serving to let him do other things. No, he really did not want a vasectomy either, he was wondering about becoming a mature student and doing primary teaching. Neither member of this couple really wanted sterilization despite peer pressure.

One cannot assume that the marriage will benefit from vasectomy (Howard, 1979).

'Men are aggressive'

Individual men are affected by the universal assumption that they are more aggressive than women, and this expectation colours all stages of their sexual and contraceptive life. They are expected to need to masturbate, and to be normal they should play the field to score with the girls. Men should know how to use condoms and know which girls are on the Pill. Later they are required to abandon Falstaff, that irresponsible Shakespearean lover of the good life, to become a knight on a white charger wooing his respectable lady. Then he must become the responsible family man, providing for a wife and 2.4 children. These images are difficult to live up to, and any psychosexual problems that may develop along the way are expected to look after themselves. Few men go for help to family planning clinics or the general practitioner to discuss their personal sexuality unless there are serious problems of premature ejaculation or impotence.

PSYCHOSEXUAL SKILLS

Psychosexual medicine has evolved a discipline of looking at difficulties by concentrating attention on the doctor/patient relationship and also on what happens during the genital examination. A man may have his closest feelings defended by the fear that he is not normal – perhaps not as aggressive as the average man. This may form a barrier to the useful development of the relationship with the doctor. Some of the barriers here have been described by Tunnadine (1983).

It requires careful listening to hear where the vulnerability lies, particularly with men, as the opportunities to examine feelings via the exposure of the genitalia are less frequently available than they are with women. When such an examination is possible it can be excitingly enlightening.

> Mr I. was a 25-year-old ex-soldier who came complaining of impotence. He could no longer get a condom on and had finished with his girlfriend although he still cared a lot for her. He wanted to talk about his testosterone levels (normal) and not about the fact that he had one testicle. One had been removed at herniorrhaphy as the surgeon said it was out of place and a cancer risk. The doctor asked if he could examine him. The soldier became embarrassed, shifting from leg to leg with his arms crossed. He said that he hated undressing in front of people, but he would if it would help. He was an active body builder with a handsome physique and cheeky tattoos. Something did not fit and the doctor asked why he was unhappy with his body. He replied that he liked it, but that his first sexual partner had laughed at it when he tried to make love standing up, after a night out drinking, with another soldier watching. So examination revealed that it was not his testicle that was vulnerable, but his external masculine nakedness.

A theoretical approach to the analysis of men's aggressive progress through life could range into several different schools of thought. One could look at his self as viewed by Freud, Jung, Adler and Klein, or at the more fashionable methods of assessing congruence and actualization used in client-centred work.

Psychosexual medicine specifically does not do this. By concentrating on the 'here and now' the doctor is made to listen to the patient and to what is happening between them in the room. The doctor may detect assumptions projected onto him or her and feel how he himself or she herself, reacts. It may be that the doctor is able to use some of these features of the relationship only because of his/her own deficiencies. However, to look at these separately as elements of transference or counter-transference brings risks of trying to tackle difficulties too deeply rooted in the unconscious of the patient, or conversely putting doctors under pressure to change their beliefs without the support that analysis provides. The doctor concentrating on the immediate dynamics of the relationship can make interpretations of immediate relevance and look for changes that such interpretations facilitate at a later consultation.

CONCLUSION

One can picture a man entering his sexual life and making decisions about contraception. He is prepared by his early sexual and family experiences, and is under a yoke of expectation from both himself and others. He may be able to accept and assimilate such forces, or he may not be able to cope, using such defences as denial, splitting or internalized depression.

In our everyday work with patients, doctors will discover that the aggressive, pleasure-seeking stud is a rare beast, but if they can listen to the hidden feelings, doctors will find a more complex human being. Although he may have times of uncontrolled pleasure, they will be interspersed with upsurges of longing for safety and loving, and the problems brought by the need to be in control.

When in a stable pair bond, decisions about limiting his family will seldom be based on his personal needs alone. He will worry about his partner, and such concern is to be welcomed, but at other times it may be necessary to help him to pay more attention to his own needs. Such necessary concern for the emotional life of both partners may lead to a move from one contraceptive method to another until one is found that feels right.

Finally, what of the end of his fertile period? Old father time is an archetype of the past, present and future. Men can father children in their 70s and it is less natural to cut off a man's fertility than a woman's, that will in any case fail. Post-vasectomy counselling is not as widely available as it should be and regrets can linger.

As a last insight, one man spoke about withdrawal, describing it as 'Terrible, doctor.' Then he thought a moment, and added, 'Actually that is not quite true because we used it while I waited for the results of the specimens after vasectomy. That was really our last excitement.' Excitement and terror are closely linked. Excitement is easy to admit. Terror less so, but what was shared here was a tinge of sadness for his lost reproductive powers.

REFERENCES

Adler, E. Cook, A., Gray, J. *et al.* (1981) A comparison of sterilized women with the wives of vacectomized men. *Contraception*, **23**(1), 45.

Howard, G. (1979) The quality of marriage before and after vasectomy. *British Journal of Sexual Medicine*, **6**(52), 6–13.

Howard, G. (1982) Who asks for vasectomy reversal and why? *British Medical Journal, Clinical Research Edition*, **285**(6340), 490–2.

Samuels, A. (985) *Jung and the Post-Jungians*, Routledge, London, p. 31.

Tunnadine, P. (1983) *The Making of Love*. Reprinted as *Insights into Troubled Sexuality* (1992). Chapman & Hall, London, pp. 51–65.

7

Contraception after childbirth

Heather Montford

SUMMARY

- The immediate puerperium
- Before the postnatal examination
- At the postnatal examination
- After the postnatal examination
- Postnatal depression
- Male problems

Childbirth is a dramatic event, an intensely emotional occasion. It is a time of great physical and hormonal change, and of psychological readjustment. Psychoanalysts have called it a 'maturational crisis' – a woman's abrupt transition from girlhood to motherhood, often bringing to mind previously unconscious recollection of the mothering she herself received. For the couple, it is a time of domestic and social upheaval and reassessment of roles. Such factors may have a profound effect on sexual feelings, which providers of contraception need to understand if they are to meet fully their patients' individual needs.

THE IMMEDIATE PUERPERIUM

As with any major event, the immediate effect of childbirth is one of shock; in this case usually succeeded by a need to care for and bond with a new baby. The woman's ability to cope with the experience will depend on several important factors, namely the physical and psychological severity of the event itself, her personality and past experience, the fulfilment or otherwise of her expectations, and on the relationship she has with her partner.

The joy, happiness and sense of achievement in the birth of the baby may be inhibited by recent memories of traumatic delivery, a painful perineum, difficulties with breast feeding or postnatal depression. Sexual matters seem an irrelevance. Several studies have shown that women experience a marked reduction in sexual activity and enjoyment in the third trimester and for up to three months postpartum. This may be nature's way of ensuring the maximum preservation of the infant by giving it the mother's undivided attention during the most vulnerable period of its life. Such a view is borne out by the tradition of primitive societies that the newly delivered woman remains with the other women until the baby is seen to thrive. In some races and some religions sexual intercourse is forbidden until the lochia ceases, or while breast feeding continues, although these tend by inference to be polygamous societies.

Since the advent of medical methods of contraception in the 1960s, it has been the practice to offer contraceptive advice to women on the postnatal wards. As time spent in hospital has become less, this advice is sometimes offered within hours of delivery! It is hardly surprising therefore that the presence of the well-meaning family planning nurse or doctor is often greeted with hostility, ribaldry, mirth or at best polite interest. Such responses may be reinforced by the attitude of the ward sister who may resent such a visitor as being disturbing to 'my mothers'. Such an attitude is understandable since it may be difficult for some midwives to really appreciate the importance of family planning, having devoted their whole life to the production of healthy babies.

At this stage the family planning adviser is often seen as an intruder and rarely as the one with whom the patient can share her anxieties about the delivery or her concerns for the future. Nevertheless, some information about when it is considered safe to resume sexual intercourse, where to obtain contraception and how to use it is obviously desirable, if only to be referred to when the woman herself feels ready to consider sexual matters. Verbal information will need to be backed up by written information in the form of leaflets, and supplies of condoms may be given. If contraceptive pills are prescribed then written instructions on when and how to begin must be included, as much that is said during those first few days is probably not taken in or not remembered, and the woman's preoccupation with other matters needs to be respected.

When the delivery is known to have been traumatic in physical terms, when the baby is not thriving or has died, or when an abnormal baby has been born, a particularly sensitive approach to discussion of contraception will be needed. The woman's pain and distress or anger at what has happened may be hard for the family planning adviser to bear, and it may be tempting to avoid counselling such a woman with the excuse that she needs help in coping with her misfortune rather than consideration of her sexual activity in the future. And yet, these are often the women who need the most help, for to treat them differently may only increase their feelings of isolation and abnormality. They may have considerable anxieties about when to embark on a pregnancy again, and even at the height of their grief they may be looking forward in their mind. Time needs to be spent in allowing the woman to share her grief, while acknowledging with her that her need for comfort and closeness with her partner could lead to sexual activity. She may need encouragement to allow herself to consider sexual pleasure, especially where there are feelings of guilt or blame. Time spent exploring her anxieties at this stage may allow natural healing to begin to take place.

Mrs T.'s baby had died shortly after birth. No abnormality of the baby had been expected antenatally. The family family planning doctor saw Mrs T. through the glass door of the single room she had been given, away from the ward full of flowers and babies. She was dressed and waiting to go home. The doctor resisted the temptation to pass her by. She sat on the bed beside the patient, and after comforting her for a few minutes she asked gently about contraception. 'I used to take the Pill but they think the baby had a tumour. Could it have been . . . ?' She faltered. The doctor rifled through the notes. The postmortem report was not yet available and with difficulty, in the absence of proper information, the doctor tried to reassure her. 'Perhaps I'll take the Pill then,' said the patient. 'But I'll wait till my postnatal.' The doctor who was still looking at the notes said, 'You'll be sure to go won't you, because I see your last cervical smear showed a few abnormal cells and you should have it repeated.' There was a silence. The doctor looked up. Mrs T. sat very still her eyes brimming with tears. The doctor, with a flash of insight said, 'You think you gave the baby cancer, don't you?' As the tears fell, the doctor comforted her, knowing that she could now offer reassurance with confidence as she knew the real cause of Mrs T.'s anxiety. 'So it's all right to use the Pill again? These abnormal cells – it's to do with sex, isn't it?'

Leaving Mrs T. after further discussion and reassurance, the doctor felt conscious of grief shared and explanations given. She felt fairly confident that in time the patient would recover from her loss, and that perhaps longstanding psychosexual unhappiness had been avoided.

Another important group of women are those who have no current partner because the pregnancy was the result of a casual encounter or because death or separation has occurred since the baby was conceived. While for some contraception will be unnecessary, others may find themselves at risk, often because of a need for loving and closeness and because of a need to regain their own self-esteem. An offer of contraceptive advice may be a means of paying tribute to these needs and of giving her permission to enjoy her own sexual feelings despite feelings of guilt or blame. In all these situations it may be difficult not only for the family planning adviser to share the patient's feelings, but she may be tempted to allow her own attitudes and judgement to intervene, especially if the patient's experience seems to mirror her own experience in some way. The temptation to discuss personal experience must be resisted since, as in all professional consultations, it is the patient's feelings and not the doctor's that must be understood. To discuss the doctor's experience can only detract from that.

BEFORE THE POSTNATAL EXAMINATION

Nowadays it is accepted for couples to resume intercourse once the lochia has diminished and the perineum has healed. Therefore, from the contraceptive point of view, the postnatal visit at six weeks may be too late. Most studies have shown that between a third and a half of women will have had intercourse before the postnatal visit (Frolich *et al.*, 1990). The earliest potential fertile ovulation has been shown to take place around the end of the fourth week, although considerably later in fully lactating women (Guillebaud, 1988).

Clearly, contraception is needed to prevent an unplanned pregnancy occurring from the fourth week onwards, and for women who have been unable to accept advice on the postnatal ward, or who are unable or unmotivated to visit their GP or family planning clinic, other provision needs to be available. The opportunity for discussion with the district mdiwife up to the tenth day, and later with the health visitor, can be of great value. By this time, and in the privacy of her own home, she may be better able to make decisions for herself. She is sufficiently removed from the event to allow 'debriefing'. Although defined literally as the giving of a report, debriefing has also been described as the process by which a person is allowed to relive an experience with someone else in order to make sense of it. If a woman is allowed to relive her experience of childbirth with another person she may be able to put into words feelings about the experience that she had not consciously realized that she had. If these feelings can be shared and understood she may be able to relinquish them.

The health visitor will have seen how she is coping with the baby, and will probably have had a chance to observe her relationship with her partner and with other members of the family. She may well have some insight into the future family intentions of the woman and her partner. Either sheaths or the contraceptive pill (the progestogen-only pill if she is breast feeding) will probably be the most medically appropriate methods at this stage, but as always, a balance must be sought between what is medically advisable and the woman's preferred method, or indeed whether she wishes to use contraception at all. To help her with this decision, the family planning training of health visitors and midwives is very important.

The early postnatal weeks are a time of great potential for helping the woman with a chaotic lifestyle (see Chapter 1). If it is possible for the woman to use some form of contraception and thus provide a breathing space before the next pregnancy, it can be the first stage in helping her to take some control over her own life. However, the subject has to be raised with great tact as the woman may feel that she is being coerced by heavy-handed people in authority. The idea of birth spacing is usually more acceptable than contraception. It is also important to explore and value any fears and mythical beliefs about the methods that she may have.

Linda's flat was on the seventh floor. As usual the lift was broken. The health visitor, out of breath and struggling to be heard against the loud barking of the Alsatian that greeted her arrival, turned off the television herself. Linda was nursing the new baby born four weeks before. One-year-old Gavin tottered unsteadily among the debris of plastic toys holding a feeding bottle in his mouth by the teat. Three-year-old Tracey had opened the door; 'Couldn't get her to nursery,' said Linda. Paul, Linda's husband, appeared briefly in the doorway. 'I'm off then.' The health visitor groaned inwardly: so he was still here! Away from home for long periods doing 'a bit of this and that' she had assumed he was away for a while, long enough perhaps to get Linda down to the doctor's for her postnatal check. She would have to raise the subject of contraception. Had Linda thought about it? Linda's eyes glazed as she rocked the baby to and fro. 'He likes kids, anyway they make you feel special don't they?' The health visitor understood how she felt. What was there to feel special about in Linda's life except for having children; what choices did she have? Her step-father had thrown her out when she found she was pregnant the first time, even though she had lost that baby. Getting pregnant again and marrying Paul was the only bit of security she knew, but Paul only seemed to care when there was a new baby around. But Linda could barely cope as things were. 'Couldn't you do with a break, Linda? Get to meet the other mums here, and make a bit of life for yourself?' Linda looked doubtful. 'I don't want no injections, they make you sterile. I've seen the leaflet.' 'Not permanently,' said the health visitor. 'And I can't take the Pill, never could remember anyhow, and he won't use nothing.' 'What about a coil? If I took you down to the clinic you could have one put in straight

away and then when you want another baby, have it
taken out again.' 'You mean it doesn't have to stay in
five years? But I'm not sure I want something inside me
all the time.' 'You had the baby inside. The coil's just
there until the next baby.' Linda looked interested. Here
was someone saying she could have another baby if she
wanted to. 'I wouldn't mind for a bit . . . we could do
with a bit of peace around here.'

The health visitor hoped that the doctor would agree to put a coil
in with the baby only four weeks old. At least the lochia had stopped
and, fortunately, Linda had no record of pelvic infection. The coil
might be expelled or Linda might bleed, and there was a higher risk
of perforation, but the doctor was skilled. Most important of all, Linda
knew she had been allowed to choose and even if it was not the ideal
method, it was the only one acceptable to her.

For many women, however, the commonest means of contraception before the six week postnatal visit is abstinence. It is possible
that those who do resume intercourse do so for reasons other than
their own sexual desire. Some will do so to please their partner. When
intercourse has not been possible for a time previously, he may need
reassurance that he is still loved and needed despite the advent of
the new baby.

For other women intercourse is an important part of comfort and
closeness, both valuing and being valued. There are also those women
with strong feminist views who wish to prove themselves unaffected
by childbirth. The sense that the body has been irrevocably changed
by the birth of the baby can be particularly strong in those women
who were ambivalent about the pregnancy, and in whom the sense
of self-worth is connected to their being able to compete with men
in a man's world. They may be unable to accept the changes that
have come as a result of acknowledging their womanhood. Pain or
difficulty with intercourse, or lack of sexual arousal may fuel their
anger and resentment and be a potent cause of psychosexual problems
in the future.

AT THE POSTNATAL EXAMINATION

The postnatal examination, usually at six weeks, is considered by
the most practical as a sort of MOT test (the obligatory government

safety check on the mechanical workings of one's car), to ensure that all parts are working properly again. Others may consider it as the secular equivalent of the Churching of Women – the Anglican ceremony of thanksgiving for having safely survived the perils of childbirth and the recognition that the woman is now ready to be received back into the community. Likewise, it may be seen as a 'rite of passage', the moment when she returns from the process of childbearing to ordinary life (Raphael-Leff, 1991).

In the past, couples were advised against resuming intercourse until this six week postnatal check by the doctor, although there were always a few rebels who broke the rule. The doctor was looked to as the authority who would proclaim the woman as ready to resume normal life. To a large extent, this is still the case. Some women like to feel that intercourse is prohibited until after the postnatal visit, for it is easier to refuse for good medical reasons rather than because she does not want it. For her partner, too, it may be easier to accept the sense of exclusion if it is felt to be for medical reasons. Although it is easy to give permission for intercourse, perhaps the woman who feels strongly that it is prohibited should be allowed to quote medical authority if she wants to do so.

It is sad that few hospitals now support postnatal family planning clinics and the opportunity to return to the place where the baby was born is seldom available. At such a visit the woman could show off the baby, have her new status as mother recognized and discuss her delivery, even though it might be with a doctor whose only knowledge of the delivery was from the notes. Some women will delay or postpone their postnatal examination, thereby indicating perhaps an unconscious wish to postpone entry into normal, and in particular, sexual life. Or it may be that they fear that they might fail the test of official recognition as a fully fledged mother. On the other hand, the woman who fails to attend altogether may be indicating her wish to guard her privacy and assume total responsibility for herself again. She will happily resume intercourse, using her old cap or having started herself on as old supply of Pills.

Among the socially deprived, poor attendance at postnatal examinations is frequent. Such default is often attributed to fecklessness but this is not often the case and may be for purely logistical reasons such as difficulties with transport, especially where there are other children who cannot be left at home. Equally it may be a deliberate rebellion against authority where the doctor is seen as someone imposing her view on how many children the woman should have or how they should be spaced. Sometimes such rebellion is not recognized as such by the patient, who will blame the practical difficulties for her non-attendance. Even if domiciliary help is offered she is likely to be out when the doctor calls (see Chapter 1).

Those with poor self-esteem also tend to be among the patients who find it difficult to attend for routine postnatal and other medical appointments. It is as if they do not feel they have the right to the attention implicit in such routine care. At the same time it is difficult for them to believe that planning is possible in view of their chaotic lifestyle so far. They find it difficult to believe that professional people will heed their views and they can make a choice only when they feel their choice will be listened to.

The postnatal examination is in the first instance an examination of the woman's physical health. Routine questions about her general wellbeing, lactation, duration of lochia and healing of the perineum will be asked as a matter of course. Details of the delivery may need to be discussed. Blood pressure and weight are checked and pelvic organs examined. However, the postnatal examination is far more than this. It is also an examination of her psychological health and of how she is coping with the 'maturational crisis' she has undergone. More may be revealed about her feelings from her general appearance and manner than from her answers to the doctor's questions; feelings that must first be explored before a decision about contraception can be reached. Sometimes her anxieties are not fully expressed until the genital parts are examined, and if the doctor can combine the necessary physical examination with psychosomatic listening and observation it can be very fruitful (Tunnadine, 1970). This is a moment when patients may be able to get in touch with and share their feelings about the birth for the first time.

Mrs B. stopped abruptly at the door of the consulting room and announced, 'Do I have to see so many people? I've only come to see one doctor.' The doctor and nurse in training looked embarrassed. The instructing doctor suppressed her irritation that valuable teaching material might be lost, but knew that her patient's wishes must come first. The trainees tactfully withdrew.

The interview was prickly. The doctor, although recognizing that the patient's request to be seen alone might be symptomatic of some underlying anxiety, found herself not only having to contain her own annoyance, but having to accept a rebuff to all her gentle probings. 'I've only come for a check-up, that's all,' said Mrs B. 'Of course I'm feeling tired, who wouldn't when the baby wakes several times in the night? The delivery wasn't what I expected.' 'You expected something different?' asked the docotr. 'Why shouldn't I? I went to all the antenatal classes, didn't I? And I want you to fit me with a coil,' she said, as if putting an end to further discussion. She brandished a leaflet. 'I've read all about it, at least I don't have to think about it.' Think about what, thought the doctor. A pause. 'What did you use before?' 'The Pill, but it never really agreed with me, then the cap; that was fine but I couldn't possibly use it now.' A spasm of pain crossed her face but she was already moving towards the couch. Breasts and abdomen were examined, then the perineum – a beautifuly healed episiotomy scar, but Mrs B.'s hands were across her eyes. The doctor said, 'Tell me what you think it is like down there.' 'It's horrible, horrible. I wanted everything to be natural but the baby got stuck. They kept saying that I should have had an epidural but I didn't want it and I didn't want to be cut. Stitching me up was even worse; there were all these people in the room. I don't think I'll have a coil fitted today, I'll come back later.' 'When I put my fingers inside you, can you tell me what it feels like?' Subtly the doctor was putting Mrs B. back in charge of herself. 'Then you can decide what method of contraception it's going to be. You might like to go back to the cap after all.' With the doctor's help Mrs B. was able to recognize with astonishment how normal her vagina felt, and even managed to insert a new cap.'Actually,' said Mrs B. 'I think I would like a coil. It's possible to be a bit more spontaneous isn't it?' She gave a shy secretive smile. She was even beginning to think about sex.'And as long as you do it I don't really mind if your trainees watch.' Having shown her feelings with the doctor, Mrs B. was able to take a positive decision about herself and was back in control again.

The importance of recognizing the distress behind Mrs B.'s difficult exterior cannot be emphasized too much. If the damage that she believed that the birth had done to her body had not been explored and dealt with at that stage, she could well have continued with pain and possibly sexual difficulties for months or even years. As it was, the time taken to help her explore her own vagina and her feelings about it was time well spent. Such a patient might find it extremely difficult to pluck up the courage to come specifically to ask for help with a sexual problem, and the emotional pain would be more likely to become fixed on her perineum as time went by, even possibly leading to requests for surgical treatment. Thoughtful handling of the contraceptive consultation and a brief body/mind approach to the genital area can prevent much future distress.

AFTER THE POSTNATAL EXAMINATION

Just as contraceptive advice at six weeks may be too late to prevent pregnancy in some women, for others it will be too early to find a method of contraception that will suit. Particularly when intercourse has not been resumed, the woman's change in feelings about her sexuality may not be apparent. As always, unless her feelings are understood her contraceptive needs are unlikely to be met.

An appointment three months after the postnatal visit is usually given to check the coil or give further supplies of contraceptive pills. For physical reasons, the method chosen may be no longer appropriate. Bleeding with a coil or with the injectable contraceptive may be unacceptable, and a decision to stop breast feeding may mean a change from the progestogen-only to the combined Pill. However, now that physical healing has taken place, lactation well established or stopped, the baby often sleeping through the night so that tiredness is less, it can be a time when emotional problems and anxieties may be revealed. Tobert has described some of the feelings that can occur after the birth of a baby, and which may present with psychosexual problems such as loss of libido (Tobert, 1983). The woman may have strong feelings of pain, rage, humiliation or disappointment about her delivery. These feelings can be especially acute for the woman whose delivery has been with the use of forceps or by caesarian section, so that the hoped-for natural delivery has not been possible. Feelings of damage to the body may have been reinforced by insensitive words at the postnatal examination such as 'of course you have not been stitched up too tight; you could drive a cart and horses through there.'

For some women who have found the experience of childbirth intolerable, and the experience of looking after a small baby almost beyond their capacities, the fear of further pregnancy may not only dampen any sexual drive but make contraceptive choice extremely difficult. No method is ever considered safe enough, and for some even the use of several methods at the same time does not give them a feeling of security.

Tobert has also described those women for whom all the physical and emotional functions of femininity are intolerable. Painful menstruation, premenstrual tension and frigidity are succeeded by difficult pregnancy and delivery. Later there may be a demand for sterilization, hysterectomy or relief from the unbearable symptoms of the menopause. Often referring to their mother or grandmother as having suffered in the same way, their femininity is seen as an unhappy heirloom handed down through the generations.

Many of us have difficulty in accepting our own parents as sexually active people and some women may have difficulty accepting their own sexuality now that they too are mothers. There is another group of women for whom the experience of having their own baby brings an 'echo of the past' (Tobert, 1987).That is, they are reminded of themselves as babies or of other babies in their life. The episode may be very varied and is specific for each individual woman. Sometimes the memory may be of past sexual abuse and disclosure to a sensitive person around the time of the birth of their own baby is not uncommon. Sometimes the memory is of the death or illness of a sibling, as in the following case.

Mrs A. took the progestogen-only Pill while she was breast feeding her second child but was advised to change to the combined Pill when she began to wean him. She now had a girl and a boy and felt her family was complete. She was already working part-time. Before her first pregnancy she had taken the combined

Pill and again between the children, but now it did not seem to suit her. She had been back to the doctor several times with minor complaints and tried different brands. This time she asked to be fitted with a cap. The doctor noticed that Mrs A. seemed very anxious and asked a lot of questions during cap fitting. She wondered whether Mrs A. was worried about choosing a less effective method, having said she wanted no more children, or whether perhaps she really did want more children and was hoping 'to make a mistake', but she kept these thoughts to herself and listened.

'Can the cap do any damage? How long does it take the Pill to get out of your system? Should I have another cervical smear?' Instead of offering reassurance, the doctor said, 'You seem to be rather worried about yourself.' 'It's only since my son was born. It's all so silly really, but I feel I've got to keep myself healthy for them. I suppose it all goes back to when my little brother was born. My mother was a long time in hospital with him. I don't really know what was wrong, but I know she nearly died. I was only four but I still remember it.'

Did Mrs A. think that what had happened to her own mother might happen to her, or was it the frightened child of four within her that the doctor was reassuring?

The doctor shared these thoughts with the patient, thoughts which had been provoked by the patient's remarks and were therefore more relevant than her previous ideas about reliability, and after a moment or two Mrs A. said, 'I think I'll try just one more Pill. There's no reason at all why I shouldn't. I was perfectly happy on it before and I really don't want to risk getting pregnant again.' Two months later, having shared her anxieties with the doctor, Mrs A. had settled happily on the Pill and all was well.

In this case the experience of the birth of her son reawakened memories and feelings in Mrs A. from her early childhood. In some women the feelings may come from the deepest levels of the unconscious, and may be so traumatic that serious psychological upset can occur. However, in many women such as Mrs A. the memory can easily be dealt with once it is put it into words, and the doctor who can assist in that process has a great deal to offer.

POSTNATAL DEPRESSION

Family planning doctors find, whether they like it or not, that they are often dealing with deep and difficult emotions. In the same way that much bereavement counselling may go on in family planning consultations, so it is a time when depression may first be noticed. It has been suggested that some degree of depression, at least that described as the 'baby blues', is a normal and healthy adaptive aspect of the transition involved in becoming a mother (Gulbrandsen, 1992). More long-lasting depression is often missed and the degree of disorder may be hard to assess. The family planning doctor, whether in general practice or in a clinic, needs to look carefully for signs of clinical depression as the patient may not complain spontaneously. The routine visit for a repeat prescription for contraception is an important opportunistic moment for screening for such illness.

MALE PROBLEMS

While childbirth is an experience of women, its effect on their partners should not be forgotten. From the moment the woman shows the first physical signs of pregnancy it is clear that the baby belongs to her and that she is its mother. The man who has no such evidence that he is the father has to cope with the emotional changes that fatherhood entails. In extreme cases this may lead to denial or rejection of parenthood and to a break-up of the relationship. Acknowledgement of his part in the pregnancy may be provided by attendance at antenatal classes and at the birth. However, diminished sexual response by the woman because of early symptoms of pregnancy such as tiredness, sickness and discomfort may increase his already present feelings of envy, resentment or rivalry of the growing baby, and be further reinforced by the mother's preoccupation with the baby once it is born.

Fears of damage to the fetus by either partner may result in sexual withdrawal. There may be an enforced period of abstinence due to threatened miscarriage or risk of dislodging a long-awaited pregnancy. Sexual dysfunction in the male such as impotence or premature ejaculation may result and may be further exacerbated after delivery when contraception is needed and sheaths are considered the method of choice. Alternatively, fear of damage to the fetus may be given as an acceptable excuse by the man who lacks sexual desire for his wife's burgeoning and, to him, unattractive body.

The male fantasy of a mother's purity and sexual innocence is not confined to those whose cultural and religious upbringing has held the Virgin Mother as an object of worship, but is an acknowledged phase of early childhood development. The first awareness by the man of his partner's becoming a mother can re-awaken this fantasy and be an unconscious reason for sexual withdrawal.

The modern practice for the father to witness the birth of his child may be an intensely fulfilling experience making up for the physical changes of pregnancy which the father is denied, and allowing the couple to feel they have shared equally in the event. For some men, however, the experience may be traumatic and if this is not recognized and understood, psychological problems may ensue. As with women, these men may need to be 'debriefed', to relive their experience with another person so that their fears and fantasies may be explored and understood. One man spoke of his horror at so much blood and mess, and his terrible feelings of guilt that he himself had caused it. Another that he feared that sexual intercourse could only damage his wife more. One man who had fainted as the baby's head emerged felt his penis would be forever lost in the huge and gaping vagina. Yet another, that his wife's vagina was now stitched so tight that if he tried to enter her his penis would break. In contraceptive counselling such fear of damage to the woman or her partner may be expressed as fears of damage by the method itself, and reason for the fear will need to be fully explored before a satisfactory contraceptive decision can be reached.

Problems in the male partner after childbirth may have a significant influence on the quality of the couple's sexual relationship. These problems may be caused by many different factors, some of which will not be fully conscious. A study of the doctor/patient relationship may provide a clue to the problem. Sometimes the couple are unable to express their feelings openly because of anger or fear of hurting each other. For the family planning doctor the problems may be expressed as difficulties with contraception, or the disturbed sexual relationship may make contraceptive decisions difficult. Where problems in the male partner are acknowledged or suspected, an offer to see him or the couple together can be helpful.

CONCLUSION

After childbirth a contraceptive choice must be made as few women will want to risk another pregnancy immediately. As always, that choice will rest on the balance between what is medically appropriate and the emotional factors involved.

The experience of childbirth exerts profound changes, both physically and mentally. The doctor providing contraceptive care is in a unique position to observe these changes, which in most cases will be part of a healthy maturational process but which may have an important effect on the choice of contraceptive method and its efficient use.

REFERENCES

Frolich, E.P., Herz, C., van der Merwen, F.J. *et al.* (1990) Sexuality during pregnancy and early puerperium and its perception by the pregnant and puerperal woman. *Journal of Psychosomatic Obstetrics and Gynaecology*, **11**(1), 73–80.

Guillebaud, J. (1988) Contraception and sterilization in the puerperium, in *Textbook of Obstetrics* (eds. A.C. Turnbull and J. Chamberlain), Churchill Livingstone, Edinburgh.

Gulbrandsen, A.L. (1992) Adaptive aspects of postpartum depression, in *Reproductive Life: Advances in Research in Psychosomatic Obstetrics* and Gynaecology (eds. K. Wijma, and B. von Schoultz), Parthenon Publishing, Carnforth, England.

Raphael-Leff, J. (1991) *Psychological Processes of Childbearing*, Chapman & Hall, London.

Tobert, A. (1983) Sexual difficulty after childbirth, in *The Practice of Psychosexual Medicine* (ed. K. Draper), J. Libbey, London.

Tobert, A. (1987) The then and there in the patient's life, in *Introduction to Psychosexual Medicine*, (ed. R. Skrine), Chapman & Hall, London.

Tunnadine, P. (1970) *Contraception and Sexual Life*, Tavistock Publications, London.

8

The sexual needs of people with disabilities

Elaine Cooper

SUMMARY

- Emotional needs
- Physical needs
- Contraceptive needs

Doctors are often diffident when dealing with matters relating to sexuality and disability. The two words do not sit comfortably together. So where does the unease arise? Is it due to some uncertainty in the doctor as to how to cope with what seem to be major problems, and to the difficulty in adapting well tried techniques and skills to meet new and less familiar situations? Perhaps the problems are just too overwhelming. On the other hand, the sense of unease may stem from preconceived ideas held by the doctor which relate to society's view that 'disabled people do not do that sort of thing, or if they do they shouldn't'.

One cannot assume that people with disabilities will have more psychosexual problems than the so called 'able' whose disabilities do not show. There may, however, be a sexual difficulty in the capacity to perform due to a physical disability which handicaps the person. The doctor needs to feel comfortable talking about the practical aspects of sexual activity, while at the same time being aware of the interactions in each doctor/patient relationship. In general, there may be a tendency for the doctor to be protective and 'mothering' towards the patient, whose greatest need is to be allowed to be his (or her) adult self (see Tom Smith, case study, p. 117).

If patients have problems with mobility or mental handicap it may be necessary to see them on their own territory when familiar surroundings can provide a greater sense of security. Few general practitioners will have any difficulty in the home environment, but for other doctors the loss of the secure consulting room setting can increase their sense of unease.

If the doctor feels overwhelmed by the size of the problem it can be valuable to break it down into smaller parts, remembering that 'the longest journey starts with a single step'. The areas of need can be divided into three parts; emotional needs, physical or practical needs (that is, 'how to do it') and contraceptive needs.

The first two areas of need may appear more difficult and may arouse more anxieties because, if the patient is able to achieve sexual intercourse, then the whole question of the advisabilty of pregnancy and the need for contraception will follow.

EMOTIONAL NEEDS

Some patients will have no difficulty asking for help with their problems as they see such help as a right, and rightly expect their needs to be addressed. However, many find it difficult to ask because of feelings of unworthiness and poor self-esteem. They often perceive themselves in terms of the disability itself with a person attached, as opposed to a person who happens to have a disability. If the doctor also feels this way then the patient's expectation that the doctor will be shocked by his request for sexual help is likely to be fulfilled. The patient's need for recognition of his sexuality places a responsibility on the doctor, who needs to be able to see beyond the disability to the person. At the same time the doctor cannot ignore the disability, for to do so prevents an understanding of the whole person of whom the disability is a part.

The doctor may feel inhibited about making enquiries or offers of help lest the patient be shocked at the intrusion into such private areas. The doctor's unease may be an echo of the patient's unease, as both are wary of rejection. In practice most patients express relief if their sexual needs can be acknowledged.

Emotional needs usually have more relevance to people with physical disabilities who are very aware and sensitive about their sexuality. People with mental handicap *may* be less sensitive to other people's approval or disapproval, although of course the situation is even more complicated when physical and mental handicap co-exist in the same patient.

One area of difficulty for the doctor may be that of inappropriate behaviour, which tends to occur in people with mental handicap who are disinhibited, or in people who have suffered head injury, stroke or neurological disease. The question of what is inappropriate behaviour needs exploring, as does the question of 'inappropriate for whom'? While there are some activities we would all consider inappropriate, such as masturbating or having intercourse in public, other activities are a matter of opinion. A nonjudgemental exploration of the problem is necessary, as well as practical advice tailored to the specific situation. If the person has not been educated into what is acceptable social or sexual behaviour, it is very difficult for him to behave appropriately. The unease for both patient and doctor is made worse by society's attitude that sex is for the young, beautiful and athletic, in whom, for instance, considerable public petting is acceptable. But people with disabilities, mental or physical, do not fit that image, and both they and others may feel more self-conscious. These attitudes can also affect the doctor/patient relationship.

For the doctor, it can be an advantage to have an interest in the subject of disability because of the awareness, insight and expertise that can be provided, although comfort with questions of sexuality and counselling skills are without doubt the most important aspects of the care that can be provided. Doctors trained in psychosexual medicine develop individual styles, but there is a common pattern of a patient-centred and listening approach which gives a framework to their work, and the security of what is familiar. When trying to help a person with a disability some change in technique may be needed if the real person within is to be reached. For instance, speech difficulties due to neurological disease make it difficult for the patient if the doctor merely listens and encourages the patient to do all the talking. The physical exhaustion and strain of speaking, especially about stressful things, takes too high a toll. The doctor must therefore adapt his technique.

Tom Smith is in his 30s and is a professional man. He developed multiple sclerosis some years ago. The disease has been progressive and increasingly incapacitating. He has had to give up work as he is now unable to cope physically with the demands on him. The stress of the illness has put a strain on his marriage and he is now divorced. He is very distressed at the loss of his children.

He became unable to look after himself and went back to the parental home where his parents cared for him, indeed smothered him. He felt he was treated as a child. In addition to needing physical care like a child, such as washing and toileting, he felt put down and emasculated. He could not see how he could live out the remainder of his life like this.

He arrived to see the doctor in a wheelchair. The disease had resulted in total inability to walk and in some loss of hand function. In addition his speech was affected. This meant he had to take a deep breath and run his words out in little quick bursts which exhausted his energy, and he had to rest and start again. The doctor's technique of asking an open-ended question and allowing the patient to talk at length was thus unusable. Comments had to be phrased in a more direct way so that he could make short replies. The doctor needed to try to pick up on his feelings so that he could either accept or reject any assumptions made. It was clear that he found this enabling and the doctor was conscious of the need to allow him to be a man, and be treated like one, with difficult issues addressed and not evaded or ignored.

He very much wanted to utilize the remainder of his life, hopefully with a sexual relationship, but was diffi-dent about the response he would get as he was not 'a good catch'. One day the doctor commented, 'Only the outside of you is changed, the old you is still there inside.' His smile lit up and he said, 'Too right – on the button.' This recognition was very important to him. His mind was crystal clear, only his body would not respond to his demands on it. His need for independence was discussed and he eventually found sheltered accommodation where he was again able to take responsibility for much of his own life. He has since met a partner and has a happy relationship.

The doctor working with people with mental handicap may need to develop entirely new techniques. Interpretive therapy is more difficult. There is a need to be very clear and simple in the conversation. It may be that the doctor is in the role of sex educator (Fraser, 1991), and needs to explore what is really going on in the relationship. People who have been institutionalized have quite often been strongly indoctrinated with the idea that they must not have sex before marriage. They may not know what this means. If marriage occurs it can be very confusing and people often feel guilty. For instance, after a long engagement, maybe up to as much as 10 years, it can be incomprehensible that it is now all right to have intercourse: indeed it is expected. A whole mixture of feelings, including naughtiness and fear of punishment, may exist.

If the doctor endeavours to continue with his or her usual technique, he or she may feel at a loss when inconsequential remarks are made, like, 'I am going to tea with Jack today' or 'Look at my new shoes'. A new style has to be developed where the comment is acknowledged, but then the doctor is able to pull back to the matter in hand.

A necessary, albeit painful, area to address is the feeling of loss that occurs when a person has experienced a major trauma, for instance the loss of a limb, or the loss of function following a head injury, stroke or progressive disease. The change in body image is very damaging to most people. The temptation to encourage bravery in the face of adversity, the 'stiff upper lip' approach, or the rush to empty reassurance that it is all right, when it is quite clearly not all right at all, is far from helpful. The person needs to be able to grieve for what is lost and to express feelings such as anger, fear and hopelessness.

Similarly, people with congenital disabilities need to be able to express their feelings about how their disability affects their sexuality.

Especially as the teens are entered, with the muddled confusion of feelings that comes with adolescence, anxieties about whether young people will be sexually acceptable and attractive to their peers can be overwhelming.

Often when there is an accident or illness the one involved becomes the focus of attention, and the needs of the carer are overlooked. When both partners in a relationship are fit and well it is often possible, and indeed preferable, to concentrate on the one who asks for help with a sexual difficulty. However, if one partner develops a disability it is usually important to involve both of them. An adjustment is necessary in their life, and space must be given to their needs and doubts. It is a time of confused emotions, and questions such as 'What demands can I place on my partner?', need to be aired. Is the partner now seen as a sick person? How can one be a carer in the day, providing perhaps general nursing care, and then the lover by night? The changed image of the disabled partner may be difficult to accept, with strong feelings of guilt. Some people feel that they should have the same feelings as before for their stricken partner, who has changed. An especially difficult time is when, perhaps after a long hospital stay, the partner goes home. The hospital may have been felt to be a safe place, as sexual activity is not usually accepted there. When the patient goes home normal sexual activities may be expected.

Feelings of diffidence in the doctor may come from within, but are often a reflection of the patient's diffidence. There can be a strong feeling of the need for approval on the patient's part, and from the doctor's viewpoint there seems to be a need to be the permission giver. When people have disabilities there is a sense in which their body no longer belongs to them, for other people take it over and do things to it. It is difficult for the patient to obtain or accept responsibility for his own choices and actions. Such a handing over of responsibility is particularly common when there is a mental handicap, where the expectation of compliance is an everyday experience, the person being expected to do as he is told and to have decisions made for him.

Encouragement by the doctor to explore choices and to make decisions, to try, and to see the act of trying as a success, is the greatest help. The person may need to return again and again for the continued reassurance that 'it is OK'. There is a hint of seeking parental approval, but with encouragement a growth of confidence and the acceptance of a sexual role can develop, as well as an ability to make worthwhile relationships.

> Jean Jones has a physical disability and some degree of mental handicap. She would love a normal relationship that would end in marriage and possibly children. She lacks confidence. At the first sign of any interest shown in her she pours her loving feelings upon the prospective partner and her demands and expectations overwhelm him and he takes fright and disappears. It has been necessary to explore this pattern of behaviour with her so that she can share her feelings and understand what is happening. She has begun to feel that it is acceptable to need, to want and to have relationships, and it has been possible to begin to explore her underlying anxieties. She is beginning to gain some insight into her desperate need to grab hold of a new partner lest this be the last opportunity, for such opportunities are indeed rare for her. There is still much work that needs to be done with this patient if she is to have a chance of finding a fulfilling relationship.

PHYSICAL/PRACTICAL NEEDS

Against the background of emotional stress the actual physical and practical difficulties need to be explored. Doctors may feel uneasy or inhibited for fear of appearing intrusive when addressing the practical problems, but it is necessary to do so.

As with all patients, a clinical examination of the genitalia may be a moment when feelings about sexuality and other deep emotions are revealed. In addition, it is important to discover the exact nature and extent of any physical disability, for instance flaccid or spastic legs that cannot be controlled by the patient, or difficulty in abducting the hips. The patient will be aware of these problems which may make intercourse difficult, but be too embarrassed to say so. It behoves the doctor, then, to note these feelings and to overcome his or her own inhibitions. A sensitive but simple and explicit discussion of the actual difficulties needs to be held. If a couple is attempting to have intercourse then the aim is to put an erect penis into an available and accessible vagina. Problems can arise in any of these areas. For a couple with a recently acquired disability, attempts at lovemaking using their previous techniques may have been unsuccessful with an inevitable spin-off of feelings of failure at a very vulnerable time. It may be that a whole new technique needs to be developed. This may involve changes of position, making love in a chair or using such a position as 'spoons' (Association to Aid the Sexual and Personal Relationships of the Disabled (SPOD), advisory leaflets Nos. 2 and 3).

Alan Green, a 30-year-old rugby player, had a serious accident which resulted in full length amputation of his leg just below the hip. Since his accident he had been unable to make love to his wife due to impotence.

Alan was very stressed and uncomfortable when he arrived for the consultation wiht the doctor, sweating and fidgeting. He was concerned about his problem. When he was encouraged to talk he said how devastated he was at the loss of his job as a scaffolder and his loss of rugby. There were major changes in his life, with his wife becoming the breadwinner and him doing the housework. When he attempted to make love he could not do it, and he was anxious about how his wife would view him. He felt demeaned by having to hop to the other twin bed when he had taken his artificial limb off.

These feelings were explored and some practical difficulties uncovered. Due to the loss of his leg he felt unbalanced and wobbly when they tried to make love, as they always used the missionary position. When the doctor asked him why he had to do it in that position he was amazed and said he had never thought of doing it any other way. This led to a discussion of other positions and options. It was necessary to consider how he would feel if he was in the underneath position as he already felt 'flattened'. There had been no real communication with his wife about his doubts and fears. He felt she did not want to upset him, and she tended to say things like, 'It's all right, don't worry about it.' He felt ashamed of the sexual difficulty, and of the loss of his limb, hoping that when he limped people would think he had a touch of arthritis. There was a need to grieve for all the losses.

Following this meeting with the doctor, Alan was able to talk to his wife at length, and he felt they could now share the problem. He had a smile on his face as he said that they had experimented with new positions and that it was now fine and there were no problems.

In this situation the doctor acted as an adviser, offering suggestions that the patient could accept or reject. Other simple remedies such as the use of pillows strategically placed to support or hold parts of the body can be very useful, for instance to hold floppy legs in a flexed position. However, it may be that the opportunity for the patient to share the painful and embarrassing feelings is even more important than specific suggestions, for once the patient feels able to discuss the feelings with the partner they can often work out some practical solutions for themselves.

The doctor therefore needs to be able to combine the skill of listening and helping the patient to share his feelings, while at the same time being able to make detailed practical suggestions in such a way as to leave the choice of which advice to follow to the patient. Such steps as the use of penile implants, papaverine injections, vacuum condoms or the use of a sex aid may need to be explored. Such simple measures as adjusting the timing of medication to maximize mobility and the reduction of pain, or the attendance to bowel and bladder by adjustment of diet, or emptying a colostomy bag, may be valuable. It is the doctor's attitude in being willing to address these problems which is the most enabling factor.

Incontinence

An area of particular stress is incontinence. As a symptom it causes great distress as it is demeaning and often seen as immature, a flashback to being a naughty child. It is a matter for shame and secrecy. Bedwetting or faecal incontinence are not matters that are easy to talk about. People seem to think that having incontinence and being sexually mature cannot go together. Anxieties and fears of leakage of urine or faeces during lovemaking tend to result in avoidance or diversion of feelings so that enjoyment is reduced. These problems need to be addressed by the doctor so as to allow the anxieties to be shared. The relief of a young woman, telling how her new relationship was so much better because, when they slept together he wet the bed too so it did not matter that she did, was tangible.

A myth exists, even among staff, that it is impossible to have intercourse with a catheter *in situ* and this needs to be diffused. If the person wishes to use this myth as an excuse for not having intercourse then that is another problem, but a catheter does not need to be a bar. Women need informing that the catheter is not in the vagina but in the urethra, and body fantasies must be explored. Again, there may be a need for addressing practicalities like position and whether the catheter can be spigotted, or whether continuous drainage should not be interrupted, in which case it is important that neither partner lies on the tubing. For men, advice on folding back the catheter, if necessary taping it, and using a condom over it may be needed. In any event, these areas of anxiety need addressing as there is great potential for emotional and practical difficulties (Mooney, Cole and Chilgren, 1975).

Although there is a general impression that having sex means sexual intercourse, it is a fact that for some people it is not physically possible due to severe disability. Some exploration of the concept that there can be more to sex than sexual intercourse may then be indicated, and people can be encouraged to develop other skills of sexual pleasuring involving the whole body, that is, not just the genitals. Heightened awareness of other senses can occur so that touching may become very important. Such alternatives as using hands, oral sex and masturbation may need to be explored, and again the doctor may find these areas difficult. He needs to come to terms with the fact that it is the person's, or the couple's, choice that is important and he must not form a personal judgement on their behaviour. Perhaps it is worth a word of warning here about doctors who are so keen to help their patients to have a sexual life that they can be over-enthusiastic. Couples often have to be able to grieve fully for the loss of full intercourse before they can contemplate finding pleasure in substitute activities.

An important part of lovemaking is the giving of pleasure and, even if this means that it appears one-sided, to be able to see the partner experiencing sexual pleasure can be very satisfying even if there is loss of sensation to the giver. Sometimes it is difficult for the partner to accept such one-sided pleasure, but if it is what they both want, then she/he may be able to be helped to do so. After sharing the loss and grieving for it, some people are able to fantasize and recall in the mind the sensations of the past.

CONTRACEPTIVE NEEDS

If contraception is required then again the biggest problem can be the doctor's assumptions about what method is suitable for an individual. When advising on contraception, the skill lies in matching the method to the patient's needs, preferences and lifestyle, within the limits set by certain medical considerations such as absolute contraindications. Where a disability exists, the type of doctor/patient relationship which may develop and the attitudes to the disability may encourage a more authoritarian style, and the doctor needs to recognize this so that the choice remains with the patient. The prescriber will be assessing the usual indications and contraindications for the methods, weighing up the advantages and disadvantages with the patient, but it is useful to ask oneself in addition, 'What skill is required to use this method?' Is it a question of having a good memory, manual dexterity or mobility? It is vital to establish good communication with the patient so that understanding is ensured, especially if there is blindness, deafness or mental handicap. To find a way through a complex set of problems the following maxim is useful: 'How does the disability affect the contraception, and how does the contraception affect the disability? When both of these sides of the equation are satisfactorily answered, one has a possible choice of method.

Communication is paramount when working with people with mental handicap. Methods of contraception are successful only if properly used. Whatever the aim of the consultation, whether it be to help the patient to have a more satisfactory sexual life, or to choose and use a method of contraception, the doctor has to relate to the person in terms that they understand, and this may mean being very basic and explicit. The doctor may need to come to terms with his or her own unease with some of the language it is necessary to use. To know what the patient calls parts of their anatomy and the various sexual activities is essential for meaningful communication. In addition, the need for repetition can be irritating for the doctor, but it is necessary to go slowly, especially if the patient has a mental handicap, but sometimes too when the patient has had a stroke or head injury where memory and attention span are limited.

There are ethical and legal aspects to contraceptive provision in people with mental handicap (Carson, 1987; Gunn, 1991). It is important to be honest in the consultation, and to explain within the limits of the patient's understanding. For instance, it may mean using as simple a statement as, 'This means no baby now'. This author has at times been asked to mislead the patient by suggesting that the injection is to prevent their hayfever, which is unacceptable.

Legally it is usual to work with the parent or carer if the patient is under age. As they are normally the people requesting help, this is not a problem. It is unlikely that a person under 16 would be seen without such involvement, for the Department of Health Guidelines on working with the under-16s could not be fulfilled if the patient is unable to understand the implications of the consultation. Where there is understanding the wishes and best interests of the patient are paramount.

The use of contraception to help with other problems such as the control of heavy periods, premenstrual tension and hormonally related epileptiform fitting can be considered. The most emotive of all contraceptive methods is sterilization, its importance lying in its permanent nature. Personal choice for the patient is thus even more important. Major issues are raised when a person is unable to exercise their choice because their disability renders them incapable of giving informed consent. Doctors need to consider their own feelings and not allow them to interfere with the decision making. It is not uncommon for the doctor to be pressurized by interested parties for or against the decision to sterilize. Where informed choice is not possible, the ethical and legal implications will need a judicial opinion if the patient is legally an adult, as no-one else is in a position to give consent on her behalf (Chapter 10, p. 158).

For any person or couple the decision to be sterilized is a major one and feelings need to be explored. For couples where there is a disability the whole issue of fertility and the advisability of pregnancy must be considered. It is important for the doctor to be able to give an informed and nonjudgemental opinion on the advisability in regard to the health of the mother and possible risk and problems during pregnancy, as well as the continuing stresses of coping with a child.

There is a need for realistic assessment without prejudice. Sensitive issues surrounding the question of congenital disability need to be addressed and perhaps a genetic opinion obtained.

A person with a disability knows how it is to grow up and live with the disability. Some will feel that there is no way in which they would bring a child into the world with the risk of their disability recurring, but others will feel that they know, understand and are coping with their own disability, and that the risk is reasonable and acceptable, as they could offer true insight and support if their child had a similar disability. Pressure from doctors based on their views of the disability must be avoided at all costs, since it implies a devaluation of the patient's life, as if their life is useless and perhaps they should not have been born either.

The decision to remain childless by one's own actions and against one's own instinct for parenting is hard and needs sensitive handling, with space given for the person to mourn their decision. As with all contraceptive decisions, the time needs to be right. Except for sterilization, the choices are reversible and can be reviewed. This review process becomes very important if the disability is progressive as with an illness like multiple sclerosis. The time may be reached when the decision to be sterilized becomes the right one.

Ann and John Watt are a young married couple. Ann has a severe congenital physical disability. John is able-bodied. Ann's disability is so severe that carrying a pregnancy to term would be very hazardous for her. For years, in fact from the beginning, there have been suggestions that the only answer is sterilization. Although it is paramount for there to be good, secure contraception, it was also necessary for Ann and John to be able to explore the options and to exercise their choice.

Her situation was discussed and the importance of failure rates examined. Ann said that in the event of failure of the method she would find termination of pregnancy very difficult to even consider, as she felt it would indicate that she had no value. It was agreed that the injectable contraceptive would give her secure contraception and be the safest option in view of her total immobility. This method protected her against pregnancy and induced amenorrhoea which she found a blessing. Many times over the years the couple and their doctor have discussed the prospect of children. Ann and John have now decided that the risk to her health and life is too great. Ann has needed to feel that she had the choice and that she had the capacity to conceive like everyone else. Now, after discussion with her husband, she has made her own choice rather than having a decision thrust upon her by a well-meaning professional.

After some years on injectable progestogens she dreads the thought of periods again and she is currently discussing the possibility of sterilization and endometrial ablation. Further long-term use of the injections has to be considered carefully in view of the possible risk of osteoporosis, which is already a risk factor for her due to her immobility. It is important that Ann and John feel comfortable with the decision made.

A group of people who have particular need are those who are terminally ill. If sexuality and disability are difficult words to put together, then sexuality and dying are even more so. This is an emotional time with many issues to be addressed. Among these, personal relationships are sometimes overlooked. The worries of both doctor and patient over what people may think if these needs or difficulties are acknowledged can be acute. When time is of the essence people need to use it in whatever way seems important to them. Increasing incapacity and the loss of part of their life which has always been important to them matters a great deal. They do not appreciate being put on a waiting list for psychosexual counselling. They need swift and appropriate attention so that they can utilize their remaining time together in the best way, feeling free to use what physical contacts are available to them to maintain and develop the fullest possible relationship to the end.

CONCLUSION

The sexual needs of people with disabilities have been considered within the broad areas of emotional needs, practical problems and contraception. In practice, concerns about all these areas are often present at the same time, although one aspect may dominate any one particular consultation. Where an able-bodied person, if she or he so wishes, can choose to ask for contraceptive help of only the most technical kind, people with handicaps are more likely to need further help to overcome emotional and physical difficulties, if they are to be able to express their sexuality as fully as possible. It is therefore particularly important that doctors and nurses who are trying to help such people should be trained and skilled so that they can provide help that is based on real insight into the unique situation of each patient, as well as a true perception of their conscious and unconscious needs.

REFERENCES

Association to Aid the Sexual and Personal Relationships of the Disabled (SPOD). Advisory Leaflets: No. 2, *Physical Handicap and Sexual Intercourse: Positions for Sex*; and No. 3, *Physical Handicap and Sexual Intercourse; Methods and Techniques*. SPOD, 286 Camden Road, London N7 0BJ.

Carson, D. (1987) *The Law and the Sexuality of People with a Mental Handicap*, University of Southampton.

Fraser, J. (1991) *Learning to Love* (booklets), Brook Advisory Centres.

Gunn, M.J. (191) *Sex and the Law*, Family Planning Association, London.

Mooney, T.O., Cole, T.M. and Chilgren, R.A. (1975) *Sexual Options for Paraplegics and Quadriplegics*, Little, Brown and Co., Boston, Mass.

USEFUL READING

Craft, A. and Craft, M. (1979) *Handicapped Married Couples*, Routledge & Kegan Paul, London.

Craft, A. (1987) *Mental Handicap and Sexuality*, E.J. Costello, London.

Davies, M. *Sex Education for Young People* (SPOD Advisory Leaflets, Nos. 1–10), SPOD, London.

9

Cultural perceptions and misconceptions

Roseanna Pollen

SUMMARY

- Family planning and the Third World
- Political/demographic considerations in the UK
- The practitioner's attitude
- Educating the professional
- The language problem
- Practical issues
- Culture as an issue for the patient
- Perceptions of power

This chapter is written from the point of view of doctors working in Britain with patients from other cultures, rather than about doctors who work abroad. This author's experience as a general practitioner working with recent immigrants in Tower Hamlets, a deprived inner city area of London, will illustrate the most obvious problems of cultural diversity. The fact that most of the indigenous patients are Cockney, and have a distinct language as well as cultural tradition concerning such things as food and commerce, demonstrates that the problems are not only to do with racial issues. It is this author's proposition that when working with individual patients it is just as easy to overemphasize the influence of culture as it is to be insensitive. To be able to provide the best service to patients doctors need to be able to judge the importance of all the influences surrounding a doctor/patient relationship. If we are skilled in analysing the emotional climate within our relationships with patients, we will not be so greatly daunted by the constraining effects of external differences. Before trying to understand the effect of some of those differences on the provision of care in Britain, we need to look briefly at the situation in the countries from which many of Britain's recent immigrants have come.

FAMILY PLANNING AND THE THIRD WORLD

Consultations with patients from Third World countries are not the only ones to pose cultural problems, as has already been suggested. However, there is a particular difficulty when considering contraception and Third World countries, for the questions of world population and poverty are widely debated, and in discussion of these factors they are generally accepted as being directly linked. Such considerations can often colour one's view of the needs of individuals if they are recent immigrants. All the issues involved will not be expanded upon here, but those who work in the field of reproductive medicine are likely to hold quite strong views on whether population control, or a sharing of resources, should play the bigger role in alleviating world poverty. However, such views may be expressed in a crusading attitude towards the ethnic minorities, that is not subtle enough to allow personal considerations their proper place.

It has been stated that, 'In general, Third World service programmes are primarily accountable to their governments and/or western donors who fund them.. They often have demographic rather than service priorities' (International Women's Health Coalition, 1986). Thus individual needs and the quality of the service are pushed down the list of priorities, and the acceptability of a method and greater security against pregnancy are considered more important. The service can become completely impersonal; for example, in Mexico it is policy that 90% of women who have a termination of pregnancy should have an IUD fitted. In Indonesia, poverty certificates have to be shown for access to some contraceptive services. Moroccan women queue in waiting halls without their underwear, to speed up throughput. It can be seen that the needs of women and the needs of the population can be at odds when resources are limited.

A recent survey about contraceptive need in underdeveloped countries gives a broader perspective (Westoff and Ochea, 1991). The authors looked at 25 Third World countries: nine in Sub-Saharan Africa, three in North Africa, three in Asia and 10 in Latin America. They used a questionnaire to quantify the demand for limiting family size, or having a space of more than two years to the next child. They found an average demand of 63%, which is of the same order as the average demand in the USA of 80%. They went on to estimate the size of the unmet need; this was found to range from 10 to 38% in the study countries, whereas it is only 4% in the USA. However, less than half those in the unmet needs group were found to be currently at risk. (This is obviously a difficult assay, but included those who had no sexual intercourse in the last four weeks, and those currently pregnant.) Also, about half of the women in need intended to use a method. They conclude that, 'While a significant proportion of women have an unmet need for family planning, the percentage of women at any given time whose behaviour appears inconsistent or irrational is considerably smaller.' Ignorance was found to play a role in only about a third of countries, reaching a maximum in Mali where half of all women report not knowing any method.

This information does not match the prevailing view that it is predominantly ignorance and cultural taboos that prevent couples having access to family planning methods. As with most things in poor countries, it is as much a question of resources as of education.

POLITICAL/DEMOGRAPHIC CONSIDERATIONS IN THE UK

People from ethnic minorities account for a small proportion of the UK population. They are, however, concentrated in a few localities where they provide a disproportionate workload in the field of reproductive medicine. The 1981 census data showed that 3.2% of the heads of households of England and Wales were born in new Commonwealth countries or Pakistan. However, in North East Thames

Regional Health Authority this goes up to 7.6%, and in Tower Hamlets District Health District Health Authority, to 13.2%. In 1991, 23% of the Tower Hamlets borough population were Bangladeshi, while 42% of the births were to Bangladeshi women (Census data, 1991).

The ethnic mix of patients in any doctor's area is likely to be heterogeneous at any one time, and the balance may change rapidly. Looking at the most recent entrants to Tower Hamlets District Health Authority about whom figures are available, that is, for the 11 months from 1 September 1990 to 1 August 1991, the breakdown was as follows:

Total numbers: 960
Sex: 57% female
Age: 67% aged between 5 and 29 years
Type: 65% were immigrants, 21% refugees, 11% longstay visitors
Country of origin: 61% Bangladesh, 22% Somalia, the rest from other SE Asian countries, other African countries, Vietnam, China
Family dynamics: 63% were part of a family group, 9% of these families had seven or more members

These figures for just one year in one borough demonstrate that the majority of entrants are in their fertile years or are the children of women who are still fertile.

THE PRACTITIONER'S ATTITUDE

The attitudes of professionals to different cultural customs change as the views of society change. A legacy of Christian moral imperialism that parallelled colonialism has been succeeded by an agnostic, generally liberal tendency towards non-interference. Lack of absolutism has, on the whole, got rid of the view that non-Christian cultures are heathen, but not replaced that certainty with very much to rely on when faced with a cultural dilemma. Modern western doctors may see themselves, and probably most of their patients, as culturally neutral, perceiving problems only with ethnic minorities and Roman Catholics. That we are not so bland is demonstrated by the intense national debate that takes place whenever events bring ethical decisions concerning reproduction to public notice. We have not yet become, in Britain, the culture of the pre-eminence of individuality. We need to be aware of the relativism of our culture when working in a transcultural setting.

The 'I'm OK, you're OK' hands-off approach, in its extremes, can be just as inhumane as rank prejudice. For instance, the practice of burning widows (suttee) is, in my view, rightly condemned and outlawed. There are few practitioners who would try to impose their views directly, but many may imply their prejudices carelessly. Those who have enough self-awareness to avoid doing so may experience a feeling of panic because they are ignorant of a particular patient's religious customs and rules, and are anxious not to offend. The pressure of time in short consultations heightens the anxiety to establish trust by getting it right first time, rather than feeling your way by trial and error. If, on the other hand, one is very knowledgeable about the customs of ethnic minorities, one will not serve ones patients well if one assumes that all patients in this group adhere strictly to their cultural mores. The best doctors and nurses will try to develop a philosophy that embraces the compromise of individualism in the setting of different traditions and religious dogma. It is more likely these days that a practitioner will be anxious not to offend, and sin by omission, rather than by taking a superior attitude.

Jusnara Khatun registered with a new GP when she was rehoused; she was a Bengali woman 38 weeks' pregnant with her third chld. She came to the surgery with her children, but no accompanying adult, and when the doctor enquired about her husband, she said that she was divorced. The doctor was solicitous for her social welfare as well as providing good medical care for the rest of the pregnancy and puerperium. Assuming, however, that a divorced woman in this cultural group would have no sexual relationships, contraception was not discussed at all. Three months later, Jusnara requested a repeat injection of the injectable contraceptive; the first had been given at a community family planning clinic, but it was more convenient for her to come to the GP. The somewhat misplaced sympathy, and assumptions of the GP had made it difficult for Jusnara to initiate discussion about contraception. Although

> unmarried, she had a series of relationships with men who supported her financially, but it would be hard to say whether or not the arrangements were commercial. It has been apparent since then that she sees control of her fertility as her own responsibility, and the choice of method has more to do with her own feelings than cultural rules.

After a time practitioners may feel comfortable with their attitudes in theory, but maintaining them in practice is not so easy. It would be simpler if consultations were clearly confined to one subject such as contraception, but this is rarely so. The social concerns of recent immigrants overlap with their medical needs. The doctor/patient relationship is often conducted in the context of the doctor/family relationships. Doctors may be distracted by the need to look for opportunistic surveillance of young children who attend with their parents, as well as trying to support the families' social needs, especially housing. The problems of overcrowding will lead naturally to a discussion of contraceptive needs, but it is important not to let one's anxiety about uncontrolled fertility undermine the relationship of trust by appearing to blame the patient for her fertility. Dealing with so many issues and patients in one consultation can be very wearing, and it would be surprising if the practitioner never felt under strain, with a sense of burning out, when dealing with such needy families. Poor coping mechanisms lead to doctors using the issue of culture as a reason for not being effective, and lowering their standards. The support of colleagues is essential both emotionally and as a context for looking at ways of making practical changes that can help.

EDUCATING THE PROFESSIONAL

Doctors, nurses or other health care workers who are new to an area that includes significant numbers of patients from a different cultural group may find themselves faced with a barrage of folk-lore from older hands. This is not always dispassionately given; those that have been in the field a long time may have become discouraged and unreliable witnesses, passing on hearsay rather than first-hand experience. Generalizations tend to fuel anxieties rather than enlarge one's views, and most health care professionals have to learn on the job. This may involve re-learning and adjusting preconceived ideas.

Akhtar lived with her elderly parents, and her son and daughter-in-law, and the appearances of the household indicated a traditional Hindu family. A visit concerning back pain allowed the GP to observe the packet of contraceptive pills by Akhtar's bed. As they had not been prescribed by the GP, and as she had thought that Akhtar was divorced, she checked with the patient that they were in fact hers. During another consultation the doctor felt confused about the way in which Akhtar talked about her family. This confusion was voiced, and although Akhtar at first tried to maintain that she was married, she subsequently revealed her rather miserable life as the downtrodden mistress of an English colleague at work. Her UK-born daughter-in-law who had, perhaps surprisingly in view of her mother's emancipation, married by arrangement, found no difficulty choosing the diaphragm as the most sensible contraception for spacing her pregnancies, despite the doctor's idea that Hindu ritual would prohibit touching the perineum.

The commonly held belief that Asian women are uncomfortable about touching their genitals is belied by the observation that many of them have completely shaven vulvae. Clearly with this family, knowledge about cultural norms was no help to the doctor who had to feel a careful way towards the individual wishes of each member. Nor were expectations based on lifestyle sufficient to warn the doctor about the consequences of a particular course of action in the next case.

Paula was a more typical cap-user in cultural terms; she worked in advertising and lived in an expensive city *pied-à-terre* with her German fiancé. Her background was Irish Catholic, but this had never seemed an issue until she needed the morning-after Pill on the one occasion that she had forgotten her diaphragm. Although fully counselled, she had needed tremendous reassurance on more than one occasion that she had not induced an abortion. Her intelligence and education and modern way of life were, in this matter, over-whelmed by a cultural tradition that links the Pill with abortion and mortal sin.

It would of course be invaluable to collect information first-hand; our local department of general practice offers grants to doctors who wish to visit Bangladesh for a sabbatical. Some doctors take the trouble to learn the language of the largest minority ethnic group, or to read up about them. Where time is limited, it is more important than ever to check that trainees have an open yet sensitive attitude, and that they maintain enough energy to continue learning. One important aspect is to be able to watch for set and ritualized responses in oneself.

Other authors have sought to provide a catalogue of the practices and customs of all the different cultural groups found in the UK today. These are tabulated against attitudes to different contraceptive practices as a sort of ready-reckoner for the health worker. This approach is limited in its relevance to what actually goes on in the clinic or surgery, and quickly goes out of date. The Bengali people who can come to live in Britain are not identical culturally to those in Bangladesh. Both communities are changing, and the different generations will readily demonstrate the lack of uniformity in one ethnic group.

Fahema Begum, aged 19, arrived in London from the rural district of Sylhet, three months after her arranged marriage. She asked for a repeat prescription of the desogestrel that had been prescribed in Bangladesh. She was rapidly learning English and, although a little shy, her manner was cheerful and open, and she took as much part as she could in the three-way consultation with her husband and the doctor. Her attitude contrasted strongly with that of her husband's family who had been with the practice for seven years. Her mother-in-law's contraceptive history started after her ninth pregnancy: an IUCD was fitted after a termination of a pregnancy that neither she nor her husband could support, given the eight other children, a two-bedroomed flat, and her own severe asthma. Fahema's father-in-law at that time had acknowledged that their religion did not permit abortion, but sought the support of the doctor to help them decide whether or not they could put their individual needs before their cultural doctrines.

Catalogues of cultural norms not only go out of date quickly but tend to encourage rigid and even racist attitudes because of their generality. They formulate a view of the doctor in relationship with a homogeneous group rather than with individuals with a shared culture. It is difficult, unless the book is on the desk top (which would be ridiculous), to memorize information that is presented in such a format, and even harder to accurately identify the exact cultural identity of the patients as they present, just from their name and appearance.

THE LANGUAGE PROBLEM

The importance of communication skills as a component of clinical expertise has been accepted without question by the health professions. They are never more bereft, therefore, than when they lose the opportunity to use those skills because of an inability to speak the language of their patients. Translators alone cannot retrieve the loss when a cultural difference between doctor and patient is seen, by one or other of them, to prevent a shared perception of the matter in hand. If an interpreter is available much more can, of course, be done to bridge the gap. Before discussing the pitfalls and problems of different sorts of translators, it is worthwhile recording this author's local experience, which is that doctors and nurses underuse translation services because they have become so used to working to a lower standard without them.

Among the commonest interpreters available for immigrant couples are their children. These are the least suitable in my view. Either the clinician limits his enquiry severely, to spare the child distress, or, inured to the vulnerability of non-white children, he uses them indiscriminately. In the experience of Tower Hamlets general practitioners, stress-related illness has a high prevalence in Bengali children, and the role of go-between must increase their anxieties. Husbands who have preceded their wives to the UK often have sufficient English language skills to interpret. Such help for the woman is still quite different from having access to an impartial translator of her words, and there is a confusing overlap in the triangular consultation. The problem cannot be solved easily by bringing in an independent translator. Our own antenatal clinic was served by Bengali women who had been trained to act as interpreters for maternity services. Husbands of the pregnant women would usually ask them not to come in to the consulting room, for if they did the husbands saw that as a very obvious mark of their own inadequacies. Immigrants from a village culture are also understandably wary of the network of gossip.

> Sultana Noor, recently registered, living with only her two daughters, asked for an abortion of her eight-week pregnancy. She had had an affair with the husband of her neighbour, and was overwhelmingly concerned that no-one in the Muslim community should find out. She wished to ensure that none of the nurses at the hospital would be Muslim. For herself there seemed to be little room for personal feelings.

If it is hard to gauge how much a spouse's own feelings may reinterpret their partner's words, it is almost impossible to estimate the interference of attitudes from an unofficial unrelated interpreter. They may be quite detached, or on the other hand, oppressive, haranguing and bullying the patient, taking their perception of the clinicians needs to extremes. By contrast, almost complete detachment is obtained with telephone interpreters. This must surely be the most cost-effective method of coping with translation. A team of interpreters in all the languages prevalent in the borough is provided by the local health authority and they are available by telephone from their office. They are fully trained to keep strictly to translation. If hands-off handsets are not available, they will lend doctors double-socket handsets. The disembodied voice is only briefly alarming, as they quickly introduced themselves and explain the confidentiality of their service. The clinician explains who they are and what the consultation is about in broad terms. Thereafter they translate back and forth and their physical absence goes some way to maintaining the semblance of a confidential doctor/patient relationship. For many doctors this suits their style of work. For other health workers such as domiciliary family planning nurses, home visits can be planned so as to be able to go jointly with an interpreter.

The concept of health advocates goes beyond translation in a professional sense. The advocates are trained in specific areas of health-related issues as well as interpretation so that they can amplify the clinician's information and make it culturally more relevant where appropriate.

Most of the time we find ourselves using limited English and a mixture of sign language and suggestive mannerisms to bridge the gap. This is expedient and can serve well enough for straightforward transactions. The danger is that practitioners become too accustomed to working in this way, and they withhold better services from their patients. It requires a conscious effort to halt a consultation in order to set it up again with more language resources, and one also needs to explain and negotiate with patients so as to get their agreement. The imprisoning and prejudicial effect of the lack of verbal communication is illustrated by the astonishing change that can take place when a translator is brought in. As a patient is transformed from a silent marginal character into an animated participant talking at length, the doctor may find him- or herself behaving towards her in a truly dignified way for the first time. If one is consistently using a substandard method of communication with one's patients, it is likely that one will develop a patronising attitude towards them. Doctors need to work to gain the ability to use a range of methods with flexibility, keeping alert for the moment when it is necessary to acknowledge that there are difficulties and a need to arrange for help.

PRACTICAL ISSUES

Certain clinical problems arise in contraceptive practice that are general to transcultural medicine. The clinician needs to be aware of symptoms and signs that indicate a disease more prevalent in such patients than in the ethnic majority. The problems of rickets, tuberculosis and diabetes in Asian patients, and hypertension in Afro-Caribbeans are widely discussed. More particular to patients in the child-bearing age group is the issue of preconception counselling and genetic disease. Recent immigrants from rural areas are less likely to have had rubella immunization. Higher rates of consanguinity in Asian couples, haemoglobinopathies and hepatitis B carriage in those from the Far East, are all problems that require the practitioner to be aware, or the record system to be arranged so as to prompt the doctor, to check for these risks.

Training for staff to use different naming systems is available in some areas where local courses are held. Birth dates may be unknown to patients from areas where birth registers are not used, and those given on passports should not always be considered reliable data.

It is common for Asian families to express a preference for a woman doctor, particularly for vaginal examinations. This does not necessarily mean that the patient is shy or repressed sexually. Western doctors often assume, sometimes accurately, that women from the ethnic majority who are inhibited about male doctors may be generally shy about their sexuality. The same outward mannerism in an Islamic woman may be the expression only of her religious conformity, and nothing to do with her personal sexual life. This confusion has a parallel in the differences observed concerning eye or hand contact.

The organization of clinics, public notices, reception services, appointment systems and records needs to be sensitive to local needs. Texts should be translated carefully and displayed the right way up. It is an advantage if staff can be recruited from ethnic minorities. Family or address grouping of records may be useful, but it is important to watch that this does not lead to an impersonal and racist relationship where staff call for patients by their address rather than their names. The domiciliary service is an appropriate use of family planning nurses for women who are less mobile because of larger families, fear of racial harrassment or who find it socially and practically difficult to go out without their husbands who are working long hours. The home visit, by its visibility, is an advertisement for local services to neighbours and friends.

CULTURE AS AN ISSUE FOR THE PATIENT

For some patients, the importance of following their religious precepts is strong enough to allow them to ask for concessions directly.

Hamida Kamali had an IUCD fitted nine months ago. She had no problems with it but wished for it to be removed during Ramadan. When the period of fasting (and sexual abstinence) was over, the couple felt that they would like to return to the IUCD rather than continue with condoms. At this point the doctor was able to discuss the disadvantages of such frequent coil changes, but at the beginning this had not been possible because of their apparently implacable attitude towards their religion. In subsquent years, the couple felt that the advantage of an undisturbed coil outweighed their religious scruples.

More often the cultural issue arises obliquely. If a patient is in difficulties with her contraception it is often hard for her to be straightforward in discussing exactly why one method is unsuitable. This is made even worse if she does not speak very good English, and if she is not used to discussing family matters with people from another culture. It may well be easier to tell the doctor that your religion forbids the use of certain methods or devices in the hopes that she will offer something more acceptable without having to go into greater detail. Religious prohibitions concerning menstruation are often quoted as the reason for the coil or progestogen-only Pill being unacceptable, but most ethnic majority couples, too, would probably find prolonged or irregular vaginal bleeding a significant problem. Patients are often anxious to maintain their self-respect in the eyes of a professional. They may behave apparently irrationally in order to achieve conflicting goals of getting what they need, while displaying moral rectitude. Similarly, it may be easier to transgress their interpretation of religious dogma if a doctor gives them dispensation to do so. Thus doctors may be faced with a patient who has apparently come for help with family planning, but who says that it is against their religion. The doctor may be rather surprised to find that only a little more pressure on this point lands them in a full discussion of the pros and cons of various methods, with the fundamental moral question about whether it is permitted or not in the first place, left aside.

Saeeda Nessa had lived in the UK since 1983. Five children had been born between 1975 and 1983, and any space between pregnancies had arisen because of her husband's visits to the UK. Since living with her husband in London, she had had a baby every October,

all boys. She had a past history of pulmonary tuberculosis, leaving her with partial bronchiectasis and
recurrent bronchitis. Her husband, who always accompanied her to the surgery, was rather demanding and
overbearing with reception staff, and frequently referred
to the Race Relations Act if they did not accede to his
peremptory requests. The GP's attempt to discuss contraception during the gestations of the 1987 and 1988
babies were repudiated by him with the rules of Islam.
The religious laws were never confronted directly by the
GP, but longer experience of this man revealed that his
bark was worse than his bite and that the family was
not in such awe of him as might at first appear. The
message about contraception was respectfully but
relentlessly put. Saeeda finally came without her husband, but with his tacit consent, for her first discussion
about contraception. It is now four years since her
last child was born and her husband smiles wryly
whenever the doctor checks with Saeeda about her
contraception.

Conversely, a physical symptom or other problem may be presented
as the reason for not getting on with a method, in order to avoid
discussing cultural issues. A consciousness that one's culture's
general opinions about coils or Pills are held to be ridiculous by a
sophisticated westerner may also incline one to pull down the cultural
shutter.

Forida Akhtar, a 35-year-old Sylheti woman, complained
of pains in her back and shoulder. No diagnosis could
be made from routine clinical assessment and over a
matter of weeks she became more and more uncomfortable with the pain, finally volunteering that it was,
in her view caused by her coil. Her husband who was
sympathetic and attentive, readily concurred, and
although the doctor felt that the pain could be psychosomatic, she was not confident that the IUCD was the
cause of the problem. With little room to negotiate, the
progestogen-only Pill was prescribed while the couple
received instruction in barrier methods, their preferred
choice once the coil was removed. Once released from

the necessity of putting up with the coil, the couple revealed that they had never felt that the coil was allowed by their religion, and were relieved to be able to do without it. The initial choice of a coil had been made mostly on medical grounds.

As in so many aspects of their lives, newcomers to the West are in a state of flux, and fall somewhere between the traditions of their homeland and the current mores of the UK. If nurses and doctors are sensitive to the changes that are taking place, often very quickly, the patient can use them as facilitators, and thus find their own position in their particular cultural and social context. For a couple who previously believed that all children should be accepted, and that no contraception should ever be used, the experience of one years' infertilty on the basis of postponing the next pregnancy rather than limiting the family can be profound. The essential part of the learning process is that their experience of infertility is achieved with contraception rather than by geographical separation.

PERCEPTIONS OF POWER

Almost as uncomfortable as the feeling that one is trampling on someone's cultural sensitivities is the feeling that one has been given arbitrary power that is on a par with their religious advisers. In most areas there is a choice between a western and non-western doctor. Some of this author's Asian patients have made the racist assertion that they find English doctors better, and the doctor is further discomfited by statements such as, 'Next to Allah, I trust you – whatever you think is best.' This has its obvious parallel in older indigenous patients who are uneasy with modern holistic approaches and want the doctor to take all responsibility for their care – 'Your life in their hands'. Finding the narrow path between paternalism/maternalism and re-education is hard.

Abdul Miah was faced with giving consent for a caesarian section when his wife's third labour was not progressing well. He refused to give consent until he could obtain the permission of either his priest or general practitioner. Both in the event assented and all was well. This may seem immature but, in fact, how often have any of our patients wished that someone who knew them well and had authority was there when faced with a difficult decision in hospital about a close relative?

It is with the younger generation in different cultures that the doctor may feel that there is greatest scope for upsetting the balance within the family. Conflicts in families of ethnic minorities are another aspect of the profound changes that such families undergo in transition from one country to another. The doctor could be seen to be fuelling conflict by making western decadence available to vulnerable teenagers. There is really no difference here in principle from judging one's position as a family doctor to any family. The call to fundamentalism by some sections of Islam is parallelled by the anxieties of Victoria Gillick to maintain parental control. Culture ought not to be a barrier between professional and patient. Working with different ethnic groups from one's own makes one sensitive to more subtle cultural forces in the whole range of one's clinical practice.

REFERENCES

International Women's Health Coalition and Population Council (1986) Transcript of a meeting on the *Contraceptive Development and Quality of Care in Reproductive Health Services*, International Women's Health Coalition/Population Council, New York.

Westoff and Ochea (1991) *Unmet Need and the Demand for Family Planning. Comparative Studies 5* (DHS), Institute for Resource Development, Columbia, Maryland.

10

Sterilization: sensible choice or serious trouble?

Ann Morgan

SUMMARY

- A successful outcome?
- Flight into control
- Self-sacrifice for the sake of the partner
- Not a cure for sexual problems
- Sexuality without fertility
- Disability and sterilization
- The importance of counselling

In the second half of the twentieth century, sterilization has become a very popular method of contraception. Worldwide in excess of 60 million women have been sterilized (Elias, 1991), and it is reported from the USA that 640 000 tubal sterilizations were undertaken there in 1987 alone (Schwartz, Wingo, Antarsh *et al.*, 1991). In the UK in 1980, one in three couples chose this method of contraception, and in 1983 it is reported that 90 000 women and equal numbers of men were sterilized, at least a fifth of the women being under 30 years old. It seems likely that the forecast made in 1974, that in time one in three couples would rely on sterilization by the age of 35, will come true (Wellings, 1986).

At present, sterilization is undertaken once a family is complete, although previously the procedure was used for eugenic reasons. Even now, it is a very potent method of population control and is used as such in some parts of the world. At first the number of female sterilizations rose more quickly than those for vasectomy because of the legal doubts over vasectomy, but the numbers of operations are now more equal. The UK government has given financial support to a policy of sterilization in suitable cases, and the success of this policy has obvious long-term implications for the provision of contraceptive services (Allen, 1981). The popularity of the programme is such that it may become necessary to move resources from GP and community provision of family planning to the provision of sterilization and vasectomy.

Vasectomy involves division of both vas deferens, an easy operation which can be undertaken under local anaesthetic. It is therefore often quicker to arrange and there are fewer complications than with female sterilization, although it is not always available on the NHS. In competent hands the failure rate is as low as 0.02 per hundred women years (HWYs). It is not immediately effective and follow-up semen analyses must be arranged. Alternative contraception must be used until the seminal fluid contains no spermatozoa.

Female sterilization involves blockage or removal of the fallopian tubes, and is usually available on the NHS. The most popular methods are by the application of clips or by diathermy. Both these operations can be undertaken at laparoscopy. Salpingectomy and hysterectomy both involve a laparotomy. The operations for women are more serious than vasectomy, and occasionally there are complications. Although they are immediately effective, the failure rate is higher than that with vasectomy. Vessey, Lawless and Yeates (1982) gave the low figure of 0.13 per HWYs, but the results of other series have been slightly higher.

A review of the literature on sterilization is interesting on four counts.

1. It is noticeable that the total number of papers on this subject is small compared with the numbers relating to other methods of contraception. This is a surprising finding considering what

a profound difference these procedures make to the lives of so many citizens.

2. Nearly all the papers on sterilization discuss possible risks of physical sequelae, looking, for example, for disease of the genital organs following vasectomy.

3. There are few studies on changes in sexual behaviour after sterilization, and very few on emotional sequelae.

4. Advice on counselling before either female sterilization or vasectomy is minimal, although there is a general consensus that it should be undertaken.

A SUCCESSFUL OUTCOME?

It is clear from the continued upward trend in requests for sterilization, from the experience of doctors and from the literature, that the procedure is seen as safe and as having a successful outcome. In the great majority of instances both sterilization and vasectomy are safe and satisfactory operations. They remove both the fear of pregnancy and the necessity for further contraception once the procedure is complete. No long-term physical harmful effects have been proved, and follow-up studies suggest an increase in sexual activity in the short term after sterilization (Shain, Miller, Holden *et al.*, 1991).

Most patients who request sterilization regard the decision as a private matter that they have discussed with their partner. They come to the medical profession for technical help, and in very many cases this is all they need. It is at this point that there is an opportunity for full discussion of the expectations of the two people concerned, and for obtaining a medical, obstetric and sexual history. Examination is undertaken to exclude abnormalities and disease. During this interview it should be possible to identify unrealistic fears related to contraception or either of the operations, and to make a decision as to which partner should undergo the procedure.

Now is the time to be particularly aware of the possibility of marital stress, and to watch for any sign of one partner being manipulated by the other. Counselling in depth is not needed by all couples, but there is a much higher incidence of regret among those who are sterilized at a younger age, or at a time of emotional stress. These problems are considered in more detail in the sections that follow.

Perhaps as many as 10% of women regret the operation, and the concept of good care must include an attempt to identify those people at risk of regret before the operation is undertaken. When sterilization is being discussed it is wise to ask both partners to consider how they would feel if their marriage broke down, or if they lost a child, although the reply is almost invariably that they feel they could never replace that particular child. Such a reply may make the doctor feel rebuffed, but it may help the couple to look again at the irreversibility of the operation. Another approach is to enquire how each will feel when their partner is sterile, and to consider which partner might grieve least for their fertility. (See Chapter 6, p. 92.)

Even a fairly routine interview must be undertaken skilfully, for there are few other areas of medical practice where one meets patients who feel so strongly that the ultimate decision must be theirs. The anger and frustration they can feel if they think they have been denied the freedom to make the decision themselves has been described graphically (Law, 1982). It is worth telling the couple that the ultimate decision is theirs, and the interview has been set up to discuss both the correct timing for the operation and to identify any problems which may arise afterwards.

It would not be particularly revealing to analyse the feelings of couples who are happy with the outcome of their sterilization, although they are in the vast majority. It can, however, be salutary to look at the events which led to an operation being arranged which later proved to have been a disaster for the individuals concerned. In most instances, contraindications to sterilization were overlooked because of other priorities. There should be doubts over the wisdom of sterilization if the individual is young, that is, under 30 years, or has marital problems. Caution should be exercised if there is serious illness in either partner or if the individual seems not to grasp that the operation is irreversible. The great majority of people who present with regrets are those who gave consent at too young an age (Wilcox, Chu, Eaker *et al.*, 1991; Winston, 1977). In these instances the operation was usually undertaken because the woman concerned was unable or unwilling to use reversible contraception effectively. The first of these reasons is more typical, and underlines the need for doctors who are skilful and knowledgeable about contraception, and who are prepared to work with the patient, often over a period of some time, in order to help her to find a method to suit her. (See Chapter 1, p. 13).

FLIGHT INTO CONTROL

Unplanned pregnancies, particularly if there are several in quick succession, can give a sense of being out of control that can border on panic. For the woman with several small children, the fatigue and despair may lead her to put great pressure on the doctor for a sterilization which she feels would at least give her control of one aspect of her life.

> A woman in her 30s, with three children from a previous marriage, came to a gynaecological clinic with her new husband. They were excited by their recent marriage and anxious for a child. She had been sterilized several years before when she had three children under the age of three years. Her marriage was under strain even then, but she had felt it could recover if she had no further pregnancies and could give more energy to her relationship with her husband.
>
> Her sterilization was reversed but she failed to conceive, and although the new relationship was stable and supportive, she became increasingly frustrated. Furthermore, the children of her first marriage felt they were no longer valued by either parent and responded badly. Soon, she was struggling to cope with disturbed adolescents exhibiting antisocial behaviour, as well as her own anger and her husband's disappointment. She bitterly regretted her operation and felt she should have dealt with the difficulties she had experienced with contraception in her first marriage before requesting sterilization.

For the doctor faced with a patient whose mothering capacities are stretched to the limit, great skill is needed to allow her to sense that he or she is on her side, and that the doctor is not denying her a sterilization, nor is being insensitive to her determination not to get pregnant again, but is trying to help her to keep her options open. Often, if such patients can be helped to delay the decision for even a few months, they will realize that they have survived, the sense of urgency will abate, and they will find it easier to settle to a method of contraception.

Sometimes the forces propelling the patient towards sterilization are to do with the inability of the patient to take control of the situation for herself, and this powerlessness may be a symptom of a deeper problem.

A couple came to a counselling clinic with a short note of introduction. The man was in his 30s, intelligent, sensitive and outgoing, and the woman was tiny, fair and very shy. They were accompanied by four children between 6 and 12 years. The woman gave her age as 28 but the most striking thing about her was her appearance of extreme youth. She hardly looked older than early adolescence, and confided that she was wearing a dress given to her own daughter by a charity. As she was encouraged to talk, it became clear she had a very low opinion of herself and did not feel herself worthy of any consideration. She said she could not respond sexually to her partner, and then she told the doctor she had been very promiscuous in her early 20s.

She was invited to expand on the bare details she had offered, and during several appointments the woman described a brutal history of sexual abuse starting at home at the age of 13 and continuing after an early marriage at 16. She felt her doll-like appearance must have invited the treatment she had received, and she realized that she had accepted a passive role where she made no decisions. She was widowed early by an accident, and left with a family to support. Perhaps one can understand how a sterilization operation had been offered to her at the age of 22 as she seemed unable to use contraception. She had come for help now because she had met a man who cared for her and wanted to share her life rather than abuse her. During the time she attended the clinic she responded sexually for the first time in her life and her appearance became more adult. She wanted another child and bitterly regretted her operation for sterilization.

It was clear that this patient had never been able to discuss the terror of her past abuse on any previous occasion. She had accepted her operation as she had accepted all the treatment meted out to her as an abused child. Perhaps it would be worth offering counselling of some depth in instances where the patient is unusually young and unsupported, and has a chaotic lifestyle.

SELF-SACRIFICE FOR THE SAKE OF THE PARTNER

In the next two case examples, not only were the patients young at the time of their vasectomy, but there is the additional factor that with both men the procedure was undertaken for the sake of their partner.

> A couple came for advice about their infertility. They were in their early 40s, the man dressed in a neat business suit, and his wife also formally dressed. She was so distressed that the overwhelming impression was of a woman with a mass of wild auburn hair and barely restrained emotion. They had married at 18 and had three adult children. After the birth of the third child, the husband, aged 22, had undergone a vasectomy in the puerperium. There appeared to have been no encouragement for him to discuss his decision with his wife. Initially the situation seemed acceptable, but as the years went on and the children grew up, the couple became increasingly distraught. They found adoption was impossible and fostering did not meet their emotional needs. They both regretted the operation and reversal was undertaken but pregnancy did not follow.

Counselling did help this couple towards an acceptance of their situation, but years of suffering might have been avoided if they had been encouraged to make a joint decision regarding their future together when the wife had recovered from her third delivery. However, it must be recognized that it is easy to be wise after the event, and with hindsight the patient may find it easy to blame the doctor for inadequate discussion. At times of stress people do not really hear those things that they do not wish to hear, as the following case demonstrates.

A married couple attended the subfertility clinic over a period of several years. As time passed the anguish of the woman and the grief of the husband became increasingly distressing. The man was in his 50s, tall, distinguished and successful. He had agreed to a vasectomy in his first marriage because his wife suffered from a severe depressive illness which recurred after each childbirth. He had felt that she had suffered so much that he should have the operation. His wife died some 10 years after the vasectomy and after a time he had remarried a much younger woman. They both wished for children, and he underwent reversal of vasectomy.

This man was totally unprepared for the very poor semen analyses after reversal. He felt that he had not understood that the operation should be regarded as irreversible when the vasectomy was discussed. He did volunteer that he had been under considerable stress at the time, and he felt now that it would have been more appropriate if his wife had been sterilized as she could not have had another pregnancy safely. At the time he had felt she had suffered enough.

It is possible that if this man had been able to talk in more depth about his feelings regarding his wife's depression he might have been able to hear more of the facts about the operation. Sometimes a man may feel guilty and responsible when a pregnancy causes illness or suffering in his wife, and there may have been a part of him that needed to make restitution to her. Doctors need to be aware of the fact that although the patency of vas deferens can be restored in 90% of cases, the pregnancy rate is less than 50%, probably due to the presence of anti-sperm antibodies. Doctors must then do all they can to ensure that the patient understands the implications.

NOT A CURE FOR SEXUAL PROBLEMS

Serious marital or sexual problems are unlikely to be improved by sterilization of either partner, and one of the most important tasks of the pre-sterilization consultation is to identify the hopes and expectations of the couple. Not infrequently the man may hope that it will make his wife more interested in sex. One man blamed his wife's lack of desire on the Pill, and when it was suggested that coming off it might not necessarily make her better he said, 'You mean I will have made the ultimate sacrifice for nothing?' He decided to postpone the operation, but interestingly he came back six months later wanting to go ahead. At this stage the doctor felt happier as the patient now had realistic expectations of good contraception, and he could accept that anything else would be an unexpected bonus.

The operation of sterilization is often surrounded by powerful fantasies of what it may do to the self or to the partner. A man may hope that vasectomy will improve his own sexual performance.

A young plumber sought advice at a counselling clinic soon after the failure of his marriage. He complained of marked premature ejaculation and he blamed this for the breakdown of his marriage, and for the failure of several previous relationships.

He had requested vasectomy in the belief that this would solve his disorder. He was quite unmoved by the fact that the operation was irreversible, but became interested when he was asked why he felt it necessary to hurt and punish himself? This patient finally agreed to postpone the request and to attend for psychosexual counselling.

Again, here is a patient seeking vasectomy for quite inappropriate reasons. It seemed that he had a feeling that he wished to hurt that part which had given him so much pain and disappointment.

Sometimes it can be very difficult to elicit the relevant history that might suggest that all is not well with the marriage. For some women it is not possible to admit that their sex life is not perfect, especially when the husband is present. Fear of hurting him, or of provoking his anger, can lead to a bland assurance that all is well. It is likely that such inhibiting feelings stopped the next patient from sharing her problems at the time of her pre-sterilization counselling.

A very anxious and distressed woman in her mid-30s came into a family planning clinic asking for postcoital contraception because of extramarital intercourse the night before. She explained that she was married to a long-distance lorry driver and they had three children. Four years previously her husband had undergone a vasectomy. Since then she had been surprised to find she could not allow sexual intercourse. She said she had never enjoyed it, but had assumed that things would improve once the fear of pregnancy was removed. Instead, she was devastated to find there was a marked deterioration. The doctor asked her why she thought this was so, and she said she had found it more exciting when there was a chance of pregnancy. Then she added that she did not think it was fair that her husband could now behave as he liked on his frequent absences from home, and that he need fear no repercussions now that he was sterile. The doctor asked if she had been distressed about her husband's infidelity before the operation, and she said she had preferred not to think about it then. Although she had been angry, she had been so busy she had put it to the back of her mind. Recently, she had become frightened about her own lack of sexual feelings and she had drifted into a casual relationship with a friend, to see if she could respond to a fertile man.

In time, this woman recognized her own anger and the presence of deep and unresolved conflicts in her marriage, and she began to work on the situation. Her hope that a vasectomy for her husband would somehow make her more sexually responsive had been in vain, and it might have been easier for her to deal with her angry feelings if she could have been helped to recognize them earlier.

SEXUALITY WITHOUT FERTILITY

Some people have great difficulty in allowing themselves to be fully sexual when there is no chance of becoming pregnant. There was clearly an element of such a problem in the case described above, where the patient found sex more exciting when there was a risk of pregnancy. Although her anger at her husband's infidelity was important, it is interesting that she herself wanted to see if she could respond with a fertile man.

The problem of separating sexual feelings from emotions connected with babies has been mentioned in Chapter 2 (p. 29) in relation to the advantages, for some people, of the slight failure rate of the IUCD. Some women find, often at an unconscious level, that they can only allow themselves the loss of control and joy of sex only if it is somehow legitimized by the possibility of pregnancy. For others, the fact of motherhood is the central excitement in their lives and without it sex becomes meaningless. One woman described how the happiest moments of her life were when, 'They put the baby in my arms and called me mother.' When she was sterilized after her fifth baby she lost all interest in sex and could not allow her husband to touch her. Alas she was not helped by counselling.

For such women there is usually no conscious desire for a baby, and they need a reliable method of contraception, but one that can at the same time allow them to fantasize about the possibility of pregnancy. If such a method can be found their sexual responses are likely to remain intact.

It is not only women who have difficulty accepting that their fertility is separate from their sexual feelings. Some men also have fears that the end of fertility is the end of all sexual feeling and even though they may realize intellectually that this is not so, unconscious doubts can cause difficulties. It is a wise doctor who listens to the man who says, 'I just feel I would not be the same.' A degree of reassurance is reasonable if doubts about a vasectomy are clearly related to the operation, but if the doubts are somehow more vague, or are connected to his feelings about himself as a man, they should be respected (Howard, 1982).

Men can have fantasies and feelings about what the operation of sterilization does to the woman, and again these can be difficult to elicit.

A pale and withdrawn woman in her early 30s was referred for counselling as she was unable to allow intercourse. There was a long and sad history of personal tragedy culminating in hysterectomy at 28 years for uncontrolled menstrual bleeding. Following this, the woman had become more and more unhappy, had retreated into a fantasy life of romantic fiction, and when first seen, sat behind a veil of unkempt hair.

It became clear that her partner was angry and unsympathetic, and that he was engaged in a long and serious sexual affair with a colleague. It took many hours of listening before he was able to state that in his opinion, a sterilized woman was by definition a useless sexual partner, and he could see no way forward in his marriage. In fact, once both partners had identified the underlying anger on either side, there was an improvement in their situation and a marked gain of confidence in the wife, who managed to pick up the threads of her life again.

Long and convoluted counselling with this couple was necessary in order to establish the root cause of the hurtful actions and anger present in both partners. They were seen both singly and together. The fantasy that all sexuality is lost at sterilization, even if the gonads are intact, was causing a great deal of damage that might have been averted if it had been recognized earlier.

DISABILITY AND STERILIZATION

When counselling couples where one partner has a serious disability, either mental or physical, it is sometimes difficult to decide which partner should undergo sterilization. The choice is made easier where there are contraindications to surgery, but in other instances it should, as far as possible, be left to the individuals concerned. They will both need to have an opportunity to explore their situation from every aspect, and to understand what the procedure entails, as well as its irreversibility.

Women with serious physical disability often experience problems with reversible contraception, but are frequently reluctant to agree to sterilization. They see this operation as yet another damage to their bodies, and their loss of fertility as another constriction on their activities.

A woman was brought to a contraceptive clinic from a longstay hospital. She was preparing to live in sheltered accommodation after a long hospital admission recovering from a road accident in which she had suffered brain damage. She was severely disabled and unable to walk or speak properly. The doctor communicated with her through her partner who was steady and caring. The couple communicated in a unique fashion and had an active sex life. Contraception was felt to be important by the woman, her partner and her advisers, but she could not accept sterilization. It took considerable time and effort to arrive at a situation which met the needs of both partners. This consisted of using a cap, sheath and chemicals all placed by the partner after he had been taught the details at the clinic.

For many couples with a disability, as for able-bodied couples, the question of the timing of a sterilization is paramount. Often, if the doctor can help them to find a method for the next year or two, the situation can then be reviewed. Not only will the couple then be older, but other practical and emotional changes may have taken place which can profoundly effect their decision. An example of such a couple is given in Chapter 8 (Ann and John Watt, p. 126).

The care of individuals with mental disability has changed a great deal in recent years, and there is now a greater understanding of their needs and less fear of their condition (Greengross, 1976). However, instances are still seen where control of fertility was considered a priority which tended to over-ride other emotional needs of the patient.

A sad woman in her mid-30s was referred to hospital asking for her sterilization to be reversed. She came with her husband. They were living a completely independent life in their own home. The woman had attended a school for children with learning difficulties. She was an only child and her mother had been deeply distressed when she became pregnant at the age of 18. At her mother's insistence the baby was placed for adoption, and to prevent any further illegitimate pregnancies a sterilization was undertaken. The woman had been acquiescent over her situtation until she had married, and then both she and her husband wanted a child. She had felt no anger at the time of the sterilization, clearly being completely unaware of the likely consequences.

This situation is unlikely to occur today, but the consequences of past eugenic policies can still be seen. Today it is recognized that the children of handicapped parents tend to revert towards the average intelligence of the population. This new knowledge has helped to change the attitude towards childbearing by women with a mental handicap.

In 1987 arguments were heard in British legal courts concerning the possibility of authorizing the sterilization for a severely mentally handicapped girl aged 17. The case was heard in the lower courts and eventually reached the House of Lords. The arguments on both sides were complex, but the underlying principle agreed by both sides was that if the operation took place it would be for the ultimate benefit and protection of the girl rather than the community (Lee and Morgan, 1989).

THE IMPORTANCE OF COUNSELLING

It is clear from all the literature on sterilization that there is a general consensus that counselling before the operation is seen as an important part of the process. Methods are suggested and contraindications to sterilization are listed (Elias, 1991). It is also clear that in many situations counselling in any true sense of the word is honoured in its absence. Perhaps this is because there is a feeling that it will be impossible to elicit any information that the patient is unwilling to share at interview.

Several members of the Institute of Psychosexual Medicine have studied aspects of counselling for sterilization and have discussed their findings. A summary is to be found in Tunnadine (1982). This author identified guidelines which include the fact that the couple seeking sterilization should have a good relationship and sex life, that both partners should wish for the procedure and that their expectations should be realistic. This group of widely experienced doctors emphasized the dangers of performing a sterilization at a time of emotional crisis. On occasions, considerable expertise may be needed on the part of the counsellor to avoid this. Their skills can be developed during seminar training organized by the Institute of Psychosexual Medicine.

The essence of most definitions of the word 'counselling' is that the patient is helped to review their own situation and make their own decisions. Such an understanding is central to the idea of sterilization counselling, but there are other imperatives for doctors who are discussing sterilization with their patients. In the first place they must give clear, up-to-date information in a way the patient can understand. They must also share their medical knowledge about possible risks and benefits, trying to avoid passing on any personal prejudices. In addition, doctors with some psychosexual training will be able to help individuals to understand some of the less conscious feelings within themselves which may contribute to decisions that are not in their best long-term interests. An ability to concentrate on what is happening between the couple, and to interpret this in such a way as to free them to relate more honestly to each other, is invaluable. It may be possible to identify punishing or controlling attitudes, feelings of guilt and the need to make reparation, and the complicated effect of such joint interaction as mutual projection (Main, 1966).

In summary, the overall picture shows that sterilization is a good and acceptable method of contraception, widely used by both men and women. A few will have regrets about the operation, but this number is a very small proportion of the total. It should be possible to reduce the number of these unfortunate people by adequate discussion before the operation, and particularly if those people who are most likely to be at risk can be identified and offered help from a doctor with skills to help them to look at the less conscious aspects of their feelings and actions.

REFERENCES

Allen, I. (1981) *Family Planning Sterilization and Abortion Services. Female Sterilization and Vasectomy Services*, Policy Studies Institute, London, p. 80.

Elias, J. (1991) Sterilization, in *Handbook of Family Planning*, 2nd edn (ed. N. Loudon), Churchill Livingstone, London, pp. 243–53.

Greengross, W. (1976) *Entitled to Love: Special Problems of the Mentally Handicapped*, Malaby Press, London, in association with the National Fund for Research into Crippling Diseases, p. 95.

Howard, G. (1982) Who asks for vasectomy reversal and why? *British Medical Journal*, **285**, 490–2.

Law, B. (1982) Sterilization, the danger of over-promotion. *British Journal of Family Planning Supplement*, **8**(3), 15.

Lee, R. and Morgan, D. (1989) Sterilization and the incapacity to consent. *Ethical Problems in Reproductive Medicine*, **1**(1), 50–2.

Main, T. (1966) Mutual projection in marriage. *Comprehensive Psychiatry*, **7**(5), 432–49.

Schwartz, D.B., Wingo, P.A., Antarsh, L. *et al.* (1989) Female sterilization in the United States. *Family Planning Perspectives*, **21**, 209–12.

Shain, R.N., Miller, W.B., Holden, A.E. *et al.* (1991) Impact of tubal sterilization and vasectomy on female marital sexuality: results of a controlled longitudinal study. *American Journal of Obstetrics and Gynaecology*, **164**(3), 763–71.

Tunnadine, P. (1982) Personal recollections of the vasectomy research seminar, in *Practice of Psychosexual Medicine* (ed. K. Draper), John Libbey, London, p. 159.

Vessey, M. Lawless, M. and Yeates, D. (1982) Efficacy of different contraceptive methods. *Lancet*, **1**, 841–2.

Wellings, K. (1986) Sterilization trends. *British Medical Journal*, **292**(1), 1029–30.

Wilcox, L.S., Chu, S.Y., Eaker, E.D. *et al.* (1991) Risk factors for regret after tubal sterilization: five years of follow-up in a prospective study. *Fertility and Sterility*, **55**, 927–33.

Winston, R. (1977) Why 103 women asked for reversal of sterilization. *British Medical Journal*, **2**, 305.

11

Contraceptive care of the older patient

Beryl Tully

SUMMARY

- Freedom to express sexuality
- Worry regarding pregnancy
- Desire for a pregnancy?
- Age and sexual feelings
- Changing relationships
- The end of contraception

How do we define the older patient? Traditionally in the contraceptive field doctors have considered that it meant women of 35 and over, as this was the age shown in a large study to be that at which use of the oral contraceptive showed a rise in morbidity in those women who had other risk factors (Royal College of General Practitioners, 1977). The age of 35 had become, as if written in tablets of stone, the age at which use of the oral contraceptive had to be stopped. This view is fortunately changing as we realize that the new low-dose Pills are far safer for the older woman than is pregnancy and that the results of the previous research was based on high-dose pills.

From another point of view, many 35-year-old women would be horrified to be labelled 'an older woman'. With increasing longevity and health, women continue to feel young well into their 60s and beyond. Many women continue to have regular periods beyond 50 years of age. The increased acceptance of sexuality as a rich part of life, and the desire to enjoy this part of themselves without fear of pregnancy applies as much to older women as to those who are younger.

Not all women, however, have these feelings as they pass their mid-30s. Another special age seems to be 40, and for many women the 'big 40' heralds a decline in wellbeing and sexuality. If their mothers went through the menopause at this point in their life this is perhaps understandable, but other women too have assumed that peri-menopausal symptoms of irregular menstruation and increased premenstrual tension occurring in their 40s are a forewarning of change – change for the worse. These feelings can be heightened by medical advice to stop the Pill or consider new methods of contraception.

Contraceptive care of patients between the ages of 40 and 60 requires an appreciation not only of the science of each contraceptive method, but an awareness that a request for contraceptive advice or additional health checks may be part of an adjustment that the woman and her partner are trying to make to this phase of life, justly or unjustly called 'the change'.

Women and men throughout their lives have to face changes, from babyhood to childhood, from childhood to adolescence, and then to adulthood. The changes appear less for men though this may not be entirely so. For women, the physical changes are more dramatic and more visible. For men, once adulthood has been attained the body does not change much until old age really sets in, unless accident or over-indulgence intervene. Women have to cope with the changes brought about by pregnancy and later the menopause. Such changes are not under their control and although the body is not abnormal, it is not as it was before. Their adjustment to these changes affects their approach to life on the whole and to contraception and sexuality in particular. For women who have previously been in control of these areas of their lives, this phase can be difficult. Doctors are sometimes consulted by patients who have been well settled on their contraception for some time. A request to stop the method or change the method when there are no side-effects or difficulties should make one stop and think about the feelings behind the request.

Straightforward advice about the safety of combined oral contraception in the low-risk woman until the age of 45 or more can be sufficient, and the safety of the progestogen-only Pill up to the menopause is well known. Reassurance that the IUCD can often be retained longer than five to six years may put the patient's mind at rest. Someone who has used the cap with no difficulty and is now in her 40s is unlikely to conceive with this method.

For those women whose partners have successfully used a sheath for many years, a failure is very unlikely, and a request for a change of method may be an indication of some other problem. For a man who is suffering some degree of impotence, the need to stop to put on a condom can be the last straw. If a woman is requesting contraception for the first time, or after using other methods for a long spell, or perhaps with a new partner, the sheath may be a little risky, especially if she is very definite about her need to avoid a pregnancy.

If the patient is allowed to express the feelings that have brought her to the consultation, reassurance and explanation may be sufficient. However, if her anxieties are not related directly to the method, the underlying difficulties should be explored further.

FREEDOM TO EXPRESS SEXUALITY

Sometimes the fact that children are now grown-up, becoming independent and often leaving home, can give the woman a sense of freedom, and she sees an opportunity to regain her sexuality. Her method of contraception may be a hindrance now that she and her husband have more time to themselves; the sheath or the cap, previously well tolerated, now become a bit of a chore. One sometimes picks up a kind of cheerfulness and a sense that sexuality is going to be even better now. If the doctor can accept such feelings while at the same time giving positive messages about the combined oral contraceptive, the progestogen-only Pill or the IUCD in a woman of this age it can be very helpful.

For many couples in their early 40s, sterilization can be the ideal method as they may have come naturally and comfortably to accept that their child-rearing days are over. In the later 40s it can be seen as rather an extreme step when the woman's menopause is near and she is in any case at a less fertile stage of her life.

However, the sense of sexual freedom conferred by the end of childbearing can rebound on the couple, causing a change in the balance of the relationship, at a time when that relationship is in any case having to adapt to changing life situations. Some of the difficulties that may arise are explored in the next sections.

WORRY REGARDING PREGNANCY

Some women approaching their 40s suddenly find themselves very fearful of becoming pregnant. Through their late 20s and 30s, although not wanting any more children and having what they believe to be adequate contraception, an unwanted pregnancy would not be such a disaster, but in their 40s the fear of it can suddenly become overwhelming. They may present with fears that their contraception will let them down. Again, reassurance and explanation about their chosen method, or a suggestion to change to something safer could be sufficient, but acknowledgement of their fears and an attempt to understand the reasons behind the fears is crucial if the most satisfactory method of contraception is to be found for each individual couple. Other factors in their lives may precipitate such worries. One such factor is that of becoming a grandparent. The arrival of a grandchild brings home to the woman or couple the fact that they now do not have the stamina, physically or emotionally to cope with a baby. Another trigger is when patients approach the age at which their mother, a close relative or someone known to them had an unplanned and unwelcome pregnancy. Often they have not made the connection until they have the chance to talk freely to a professional person, when they may be surprised at what they find themselves saying.

New-found independence, which often comes when there has been a final acceptance that the child-bearing days are over, provides freedom to enjoy life as a couple again. In the same way a new job or entry into training for a new career makes the need to avoid pregnancy or prime importance, so couples may need to reconsider their contraceptive method.

At this stage in life a late period can be a cause of great alarm. Pregnancy must be excluded, for an assumption that the patient is menopausal is unhelpful and may give a sense of false security which is disastrously dispelled if a pregnancy is later confirmed. If the woman has been using the rhythm method or the safe period, with or without the intermittent use of a barrier method, explanation is necessary: now that she is peri-menopausal she cannot rely on the safe period as her menstrual cycle will be irregular. Women who have continued to use natural family planning or a combination of those methods with a barrier method may need a lot of education and support, as well as an examination of their fears if they are to be helped to use a safer method such as the IUCD or hormonal contraception. The fact that they have not chosen those methods before may tell doctors something about their feelings towards them.

DESIRE FOR PREGNANCY?

Some women suddenly have a last minute desire for a pregnancy. They may have felt their family was complete, but sensed that their options were still open. Suddenly it seems that they are 40 and it is now or never. They may just stop their contraceptive method without medical advice. If they become pregnant and they continue to want the baby then that is fine and they present at the antenatal clinic. Other women present with side-effects regarding their method of contraception or come asking to stop it saying that they are thinking of having a baby. For others the decision may not be fully conscious and they may ask for a change to a less reliable method, for instance, from the combined oral contraceptive to the sheath, without realizing why they wish to do so. Even if they do understand what they want, they may be uncomfortable about sharing their wish with a doctor whom they imagine to have a disapproving attitude to the idea of a pregnancy later in life.

Mrs R. presented complaining that she felt slightly sick when taking her Pills, which she had been on for several years with no problems. She thought that now she was 40 she and her husband would use sheaths. The doctor agreed with what she wanted to do, saying the sheath was a good method, but not as efficient as the Pill, and how would she feel if she did get pregnant? Mrs R. then confided that this was really what she wanted. Her children were now at school and growing up, she had often wondered if she wanted a fourth child and now at 41 she felt she had to make that decision. Using a sheath would give her some chance of getting pregnant. Her ambivalence was shown by her inability to stop all contraception, and such a non-verbal clue may suggest that she is not altogether happy with her decision.

For the doctor there are the additional difficulties of weighing up the medical risks of a pregnancy in a woman of this age. It has been shown that in the years 1976 to 1987 in the UK, the risk of death in pregnancy for a woman over 40 was 10 times that of a woman between 20 and 24 years; 5 in 10 000 against 0.5 in 10 000 according to the report on Confidential Enquiries into Maternal Deaths (1991). However, there is some evidence that this risk is decreasing in the UK, as figures for 1985 to 1987 show a rate of only 2 in 10 000 deaths of women over 40 (Drife, 1992). In the end it is the couple who must be allowed to make the choice with the help of up-to-date information from their doctor. It is a delicate balance for the doctor to share the patient's joy while providing her with realistic facts.

Some women are able to recognize their ambivalence only when their desire for a pregnancy looks as if it could become a reality.

Mrs Y. and her husband decided to stop using the sheath. She was 38 years old and her youngest child was at secondary school. She had always loved having babies and decided to have one last fling. However, the first time they made love without the sheath she was suddenly aware of what it really meant. Until then she had remembered only the happiness of having a new baby. Now she also remembered the disturbed nights, and the lack of freedom to enjoy life with her husband and the other children. Recognizing the reality of having a baby at this stage in her life she decided to come for postcoital contraception.

It is important for the doctor to understand such ambivalent feelings for they lead to apparently inconsistent behaviour by women and their partners. It will be difficult to avoid judging patients if the doctor makes decisions based on his or her own rational ideas, and that will make it difficult to meet their needs.

The question of whether it is better to use the postcoital IUCD for patients in this age group rather than the oral (Yuzpe) method, should be considered. The postcoital IUCD appears to give 100% security from pregnancy, thus avoiding the difficult dilemma of whether to terminate or continue with an unwanted pregnancy. There is less likely to be a risk of pelvic inflammatory disease than in the younger unmarried patient, and the device can be kept in as a permanent method if the patient wishes.

AGE AND SEXUAL FEELINGS

Some women of any age find it hard to ask for help which is essentially help to be sexual. The older woman may find it harder because of a perception within herself that sex is for the young, or because of a feeling that the doctor will disapprove of sexuality in someone of her age. The widowed and the divorced may have an added sense of disloyalty, especially if the previous partner was known to the doctor. For women with an extramarital partner, especially if the husband has had a vasectomy, the problem is even greater.

A request for postcoital contraception may also be difficult. It may be forgivable for the young to make mistakes or get carried away in a moment of passion, but there is a feeling that at over 40 society expects you to know better. Or perhaps it is a feeling that society does not expect you to have strong, that is sexual, feelings at such an age. Yet women in this situation have to approach an authoritative member of society for help. It must not be forgotten that doctors are still seen as authority figures. In this context it may be particularly difficult to approach the general practitioner, however good and sympathetic he may be. Indeed, this very goodness and concern for the patient can be a barrier. Most people want their regular doctor to see them as a sensible and competent, and it can be particularly difficult to expose the silly side of oneself to the person who will be providing continuing medical care. An alternative source of help, where the patient need never return unless she wants, is vital.

The acceptance of the patient's sexuality is as important as prescribing the right method. A nonjudgemental acceptance and a willingness to allow the patient to explore any feelings of guilt, embarrassment and sometimes even shame is as important as the provision of postcoital contraception. It is important that such feelings are dealt with when they are offered, for if left unresolved they can be very destructive. Such help need not be time consuming and it can prevent subsequent problems in sexual health and relationships which are a potent source of ill health (Sims, 1992).

Younger doctors and nurses may feel uncomfortable when patients old enough to be their parents need help with sexual matters. With experience they will notice that only with some patients do they feel embarrassment, and such a feeling is usually a response to patients who have some feeling within themselves about their age and sex. Indeed, some people may choose, either consciously or unconsciously, to consult someone whom they perceive to belong to a generation that knows about sex and will not be easily shocked.

Contraceptive and sexual problems at this age may be a symptom of difficulty in adjusting to the inevitable changes in role and pattern of life.

Mrs G. was a 37-year-old mother of three. Two of the children were from a previous marriage, and she had a five-year-old daughter of the present marriage. She had been trying desperately for another baby for the last few years, but all the fertility tests were normal. Menstrual problems and a dilation and currettage were finally followed by an admission that sex did not seem to mean much any more and was not worth the effort. She felt she was passing into the phase of old age and it was as though there was not going to be much to look forward to. At a subsequent visit she talked further about the baby she had not conceived, but she looked more cheerful and said she had just become a grandmother. She went on to say that she was beginning to come to terms with the fact that she probably was not going to become pregnant. She added, 'I've bought myself a dishwasher.' It seemed for a moment a strange thing to bring into the conversation, for her talk was usually about gynaecological problems, fertility tests and her feelings about pregnancy. She was not one of those patients who talked about the mundane things at home. The doctor suggested that the remark was about what she felt, and she replied, 'Well, I don't see why I should spend so much time at the sink, there are other things I could be doing now!'

It was clear that this patient had moved on and was beginning to look forward to being freer and to doing different things with her life. Hopefully her sexual life will return, too, when she can value it again for itself rather than as a means to a pregnancy.

For some women it is not so much the loss of future babies that is the underlying sadness, but a more general sense that the end of the ability to be a fertile woman is the end of a central part of herself, something which is in some way the essence of her being.

Mrs S. had attended the family planning clinic regularly for many years. Unusually, she missed two appointments and when she did appear she said she did not need to be seen but had just brought some unused supplies back. A perceptive receptionist suggested she should stay and be seen.

She told the doctor that she did not think she needed contraception now because she was 50. However, she admitted she was still having regular periods and the doctor explained that she still needed to use her cap. Mrs S. looked glum, and when the doctor commented on that she explained that she had lost all interest in sex for the last 18 months. Her general practitioner had started her on hormone replacement therapy but she was not better. Through the ensuing discussion she revealed much ambivalance about the menopause, denying anxiety yet making remarks like, 'It seems like the end of everything' and 'I suppose this is what it is going to be like now'. She denied being worried about getting old, yet saw the menopause as a watershed after which decline was inevitable. The overwhelming feeling in the consultation was of hopelessness combined with fatalistic acceptance. Sharing these feelings with a doctor who could tolerate the despair helped her to look at some of the possible origins of the sadness and to begin to accept the changes more realistically. One clue that struck a chord of understanding was her recall, as a young teenager, of the female members of the extended family, grouped together muttering and commiserating about 'the change'. Though she could not remember the details of what they were saying, there was a sense of secrecy and foreboding emanating from their conclave. She remembered the 'frumpiness' of her mother and the separate lives her grandparents led.

Listening to such accounts one can understand the power of myth and legend that is handed down from generation to generation. Perhaps this is where the art of medicine comes in, to demystify and clarify.

CHANGING RELATIONSHIPS

Some women enter this phase of life with unresolved feelings of resentment and anger which can affect their contraceptive decisions. Previously the need for contraception had been obvious, and while they were busy with the home and children, the use of contraception was accepted and had become a routine. However, having acknowledged that their child-bearing days are over, they may feel that it is their partner's turn. When these feelings are suppressed it can lead to deliberate or unconscious pressure on the partner to use a sheath or have a vasectomy. If the doctor is sensitive to such unspoken feelings it may be possible to help the woman to continue to take contraceptive responsibility herself. On the other hand, once the feelings have been explored it may become apparent that the man has a genuine wish to play his part now, and he may be happy to have a vasectomy. The worst outcome is if she stops all contraception, or changes to a less safe method such as the sheath and becomes pregnant. Then the angry feelings that she already has are likely to be exacerbated by the agony of having to decide between an unwanted baby and a termination. Such a decision can be particularly difficult when the couple are older, especially when strong religious views conflict with a realistic appreciation of the dangers and difficulties.

It is not just the relationship between the couple that is changing, but that with other members of the family as well. Parents are getting older and may need more support leading to great pressure on the middle generation. The 'what about me?' syndrome has been described (Lincoln, 1992), where the woman feels that everyone is making demands on her and she has no time or cherishment for herself. It is worth remembering that grief following the death of a parent can affect sexuality and thus contraceptive use. For some people, sexual closeness can be a comfort when they are mourning, but for others it is just too painful to open out to the depth of feeling that sexual abandonment implies.

As children grow up they develop sexual lives of their own and their parents may find that their own sexual lives are affected. Just as some women cannot enjoy themselves sexually if they know their mother is sexually unhappy, so some mothers are inhibited from continuing to be sexual if their children are unhappy or if their sexual lives are in trouble.

Mrs X., an attractive 43-year-old woman, attended her doctor regularly for repeat prescriptions of the progestogen-only Pill. At a recent visit she looked tense and complained that intercourse was painful. She wondered if she should stop the Pill as it seemed to be causing dryness. She had no other menopausal symptoms and physical examination was normal.

While she dressed after the examination she began to talk more about how she had not enjoyed intercourse for the last few months, and how she had to force herself for her husband's sake. They were both keen church members who believed that sex was an important part of the bond between them. When the doctor asked if there had been any change in her life at the time the pain started there was a long silence, and then amid tears, Mrs X. told how her 20-year-old son had announced that he was a homosexual. Despite a great effort to be understanding, both she and her husband were having difficulty coming to terms with the news.

Until that moment with the doctor Mrs X. had not put the two problems together in her mind. Now she could begin to understand how the shock had effected her ability to get in touch with her own sexual feelings. It seemed that whenever she began to relax sexually, images of her son came into her mind. After discussion she seemed easier and decided to continue with the progestogen-only Pill.

The relevance of tensions within a family to a particular sexual difficulty cannot be guessed by the doctor and may not have been appreciated by the patient until she or he can talk freely about whatever comes to mind. Then the listening doctor may be able to make the connection with the patient and they can continue to work together to resolve the problem.

THE END OF CONTRACEPTION

Some people are only too delighted to be able to put the fear of pregnancy behind them and embark on a sexual life free from the nuisance of contraception. For others, as has been suggested, the ambivalence about making the change to the next phase of life can cause problems. At the present time there is often a gap between the onset of menopausal symptoms and the moment when natural infertility can be assured. It is to be hoped that it will not be long before there are hormonal preparations that will allow this gap to be filled more smoothly.

In some instances the patient is reluctant to stop a method because of the noncontraceptive advantages it provides. If the woman finds the messiness of sex unpleasant she may prefer her partner to continue to use the sheath. It can be difficult to persuade some women to stop the Pill, especially if they have the not uncommon feeling that it is keeping them young in mind and body. Changing to hormone replacement therapy (HRT) can usually overcome this problem. Yet other women feel that the method used is acting as a protection to their body.

Mrs E. had always used a diaphragm successfully. She went through the menopause at about 52 years with few problems, her periods stopping within about six months. A year after they stopped the doctor explained that she was now free to stop using her cap, and was therefore a little surprised to find her still collecting supplies six months later. Mrs E. looked defensive and uncomfortable as she explained that she had always felt contraceptively secure using her cap but at the same time she had seen it as a safeguard against cancer. She accepted that she did not need it for contraception but could not relinquish its use as a protective for the cervix. She was afraid that the doctor would prevent her getting more supplies as she no longer needed it for contraception. She also admitted that newspaper articles about the cost-effectiveness of the NHS made her feel uneasy. Talking about these feelings with the doctor, and being given some explanation about the causative factors involved in carcinoma of the cervix, has enabled her to look forward to lessening her attachment to the cap. Meanwhile she continues to use it, collecting supplies with the doctor's blessing and looking happy again.

In summary, doctors and nurses providing contraceptive care for this age group should have detailed knowledge of the range of methods that can be offered safely. There is also a need to be aware of the hidden agenda that can lie behind a request for contraceptive advice, or problems with a method that has previously been satisfactory. The particular difficulties that some people in this age group have in asking for help must be recognized by the provision of choice within the contraceptive service, and by training doctors and nurses to be able to pick up indirect clues that the patient may be in trouble. It is particularly important that any assumptions and prejudices about age and sexuality are recognized so that appropriate care can be given to each individual patient based on their own needs rather than the preconceived ideas of the doctor.

REFERENCES

Confidential Enquiries into Maternal Deaths in the United Kingdom (1991) HMSO, London.
Drife, J. (1992) Personal communication.

Lincoln, R. (1992) Middle age, in *Psychosexual Medicine: A Study of Underlying Themes*, Chapman & Hall, London, pp. 173–83.

Royal College of General Practitioners (1977) Oral contraceptive study, *Lancet*, **2**, 727–33.

Sims, A. (1992) Marital breakdown and health. *British Medical Journal*, **304**, 457–8.

12

Psychosexual problems in the contraceptive consultation

Gill Wakley

SUMMARY

- Choice of venue and doctor
- Examining the whole patient
- Overt sexual complaints
- Covert presentations
- Beginning sexual activity
- Relationship problems
- Trouble with babies
- Am I too old for sex?
- Further treatment or referral?

Just as the bulge of the pregnant abdomen proclaims that sexual activity has taken place, patients who attend a doctor for contraceptive advice reveal that they are sexually active or wish to become so. An intensely private matter becomes one of public knowledge and concern. It is not surprising that people find it difficult to acknowledge that they are behaving in a way which may require contraception. Often obtaining birth control advice can seem like an assault course. First finding out where to obtain it, then making an appointment (and having to *wait* for it – lust and love are impatient emotions), reaching the venue, and then revealing their need to so many people – the receptionist, the nurse, the doctor and perhaps the pharmacist too. It is amazing that some manage to surmount all the hurdles and obtain what they require.

It needs to be realized, too, that patients do not *want* to use contraceptives at all – nobody looks forward in keen anticipation to using the chosen method – so that a contraceptive method which affects the enjoyment of sexual behaviour may be discontinued. As Robert Snowden said in the foreword 'Contraception is not normally viewed by users in an objective clinical manner but within the context of an erotic and emotional experience'.

CHOICE OF VENUE AND DOCTOR

A patient who is confident about her sexuality and can be open about her sexual activity, is able to ask without embarrassment for an appointment to see her own general practitioner (GP) in a clinic publicised as a 'family planning clinic'. A person less confident may need to make an appointment for an ordinary surgery session so that no revelation of sexuality is made until in the safety of the doctor's room. Even this may be too overwhelming – all doctors recognize patients who complain of heavy painful periods, cystitis, or even non-related symptoms such as a sore throat or a rash, when contraception or discussion of sexual matters is the real reason for the consultation. Doctors have to be sensitive to the clues and be prepared to enquire if the patient wanted to discuss anything else, or even to be more direct and ask if any advice on contraception is needed.

Sometimes any contact with a familiar doctor may be perceived as too threatening. A young girl may be unwilling to reveal her sexual needs to a doctor whom she regards as an extension of her parents, particularly her father, and therefore (she feels) bound to disapprove. The occasional publicity about parents being told about their daughter's sexual activity by a doctor, or even the presence of a rumour about lack of confidentiality, will further discourage the timid or unsure. This part of the growing up process which has to be kept hidden from parental supervision and knowledge, the secret inner world, this search for the separate individual self which is the adult into which the adolescent is developing, prevents the not-yet-quite-adult from consulting those he or she views as being in the parental role. Doctors, teachers, school nurses, as well as parents, all recognize the difficulties of reaching past the defences of the often sullen and rebellious teenager or young adult. Particularly if there are difficulties – the unsuitable boyfriend, a fear of infection or abnormality, failure of erection, pain or dissatisfaction with intercourse – a stranger may need to be sought out. A clinic or doctor unknown previously, perhaps recommended by a friend as sympathetic, is consulted instead of the familiar family doctor.

The older age groups may also be reluctant to reveal their sexual activity to their regular medical attendants (or their staff), but for slightly different reasons. They may not wish to bother their doctors – who they view as caring for ill people – with their contraceptive needs which they feel are less important. They may fear that their sexuality is not acceptable to their doctors, to the staff or to other patients whom they encounter in the surgery and who may enquire why they are attending. One woman in her 40s travelled many miles to attend a clinic far from her home. Married to the minister of a strict religious sect, she could not risk revealing to her husband's flock that she was sexually active and needed to use a diaphragm to prevent pregnancy. She could not refuse him intercourse, nor did she wish to do so, although she felt it was somehow wrong and sinful not to be above such base human emotions. She feared further pregnancy with advancing years, but saw her need for contraception as a betrayal of her husband's teaching which had to be concealed from his congregation. Her ambivalent attitudes had made her an unpopular patient at the family planning clinic she attended; she had managed to make most of the staff feel that they were somehow dealing in something unsavoury and undesirable.

Another woman attended a community family planning clinic rather than her own GP (a keen enthusiast for contraceptive provision who was always trying to persuade her to attend him instead!), because she wanted to be supplied with two diaphragms. One she left in the drawer at home in the mornings, the other went to work with her to be used with her lover at lunchtime. The secret had to be kept from her GP who was a golf partner of her husband.

A 30-year-old woman registered with a different GP for her contraceptive needs from the one she attended for general medical care. She explained the change by complaining that her regular doctor had told her that, at 30, it was time she came off the Pill and thought about a family. She also complained that he had not treated her vaginal discharge properly as she still had it. How easy it would be for the second doctor to side with the patient and believe that the first doctor had been tactless, insensitive and incompetent. The second doctor felt that the woman had some other hidden reason for her dispropor-tionate distress and anger with the previous doctor and enquired further. Eventually the woman revealed that she had been unable to tell the previous doctor that her partner was already married with a family of his own. She had concealed how angry she had been with the doctor for making her confront the knowledge that she would never be able to have a child of her own if she continued with the same partner. Her complaints of vaginal discharge and loss of libido could only be understood within the context of her circumstances, hidden from her own doctor because of her shame, guilt and anger.

Patients in the older group may have anxieties about whether they should be still sexually active and hide their requests for advice about contraception behind other complaints such as vaginal soreness or period problems in the same way as those just beginning their sexual life. They may need to try out a different doctor from their usual one in the hope that these clues may picked up. The familiarity which is such an asset in general practice may be an obstacle if doctors assume that they know why the patient has attended. A new doctor/patient interaction can allow attention to be paid to covert presentations, and the doctor is less likely to slip into a social interaction, rather than a medical one, as may occur with a well-known patient. Missing thyroid disease or anaemia in a patient seen regularly is a well-known occurrence; less well recognized is the inattention to the unspoken needs of the patient. The woman who attends regularly for her oral contraceptive checks may be unable to bypass the doctor's routine enquiries to broach the difficulties she is having; the doctor assumes all is well and fails to notice the hesistations or unease. Only by attending another doctor, who does not know why she has come, can she change the focus of the consultation.

Some patients hope to be supplied with contraception almost by remote control: they attend with several small children and multiple complaints, slipping in a request for 'and can I have some Pills while I'm here?' The exhausted doctor, trying to stop the children from wrecking the surgery and smearing their sticky hands over everything within reach, reaches for the pen and only half-heartedly suggests that the mother should attend for herself next time. The doctor should not be surprised when this patient reattends pregnant yet again, having taken the Pills incorrectly or having stopped them because she 'didn't feel right taking them'. The patient's feelings, her inability to control anything (the children, her husband, life) were disguised by her reluctance to let the doctor near enough to examine anything – even her blood pressure. Domiciliary family planning may be the only answer initially for this patient; she may be able to let the doctor or nurse near enough to discover her needs when her own territory allows her at least some control.

EXAMINING THE WHOLE PATIENT

Expectations of what will happen during consultations for family planning influence the choice between clinic or general practice, or between known or unfamiliar doctors.

Patients may attend a community family planning clinic because they have heard that patients have a 'thorough examination' there. On the first attendance the patient may look disappointed when she is told that the examination of that (sexual) part of her body – her genitals and breasts – can be left until later. She wants an examination of this part of her about which she has unspoken anxieties – perhaps doubts that it is 'good enough' to be shown to a partner, or that, untried, it may not function well enough, or might become out of control.

Other patients will provide clues about hidden problems from their reaction to suggested physical examinations. Most women attending for contraceptive consultations expect a vaginal examination and doctors feel that it is appropriate to offer it. Some may welcome it (as above), most regard it as a necessary evil, but some positively avoid it. The patient who always attends with a period, or break-through bleeding, or has to dash off to another appointment, needs to have her anxieties about vaginal examination explored. One patient who avoided examination feared that the doctor would be able to tell that she had had a previous termination of pregnancy, which had been arranged without telling her GP. Another was having painful inter-course and feared that the examination would be painful, or reveal some sinister cause for the pain. When finally achieved, it was found to be due to vaginismus, which was be relieved by an understanding of the 'fear–contraction of muscles–pain–fear' cycle. Insisting that the patient must be examined without noticing the nonverbal signals of incipient panic can lead to disaster. One doctor related the story of a patient who had been told to undress in an examination cubical and await the arrival of the doctor to do a cervical smear. The doctor arrived to find the cubical locked against him and the unnoticing nurse had to spend many minutes persuading the patient that she could leave without being touched. The doctor had to refer the patient onto a colleague (she refused ever to attend him again) and the history of nonconsummation eventually emerged.

Doctors who notice that they are avoiding the physical examination of a patient need to understand the reasons. Perhaps the patient behaves in a sexual way, so that the doctor feels not like a doctor, but more like a potential sexual partner. Although more common between a male doctor and a female patient, awareness of homosexual feelings or fantasies may also be required. Feelings that physical examination is too intrusive, abusive or dangerous may alert the doctor to the possibility of previous sexual abuse, or occasionally to other well-hidden problems, including neurotic or even psychotic fantasies.

Although psychogenic problems are often missed or ignored, it is just as serious to miss a physical or iatrogenic cause for a sexual problem. Oral contraceptives can occasionally cause depression, although other reasons are more common (Herzberg, Draper, Johnson *et al.*, 1971). Sexual desire disappears early in depression, often before there are many other more obvious symptoms. An imbalance of hormones can cause vaginal dryness; it may not be lack of arousal but lack of mucus. Intrauterine devices can cause dyspareunia in either partner. Spermicides, diaphragms and condoms can sometimes cause or exacerbate genital soreness and irritation. Other problems not associated directly with contraception must also be borne in mind – infections, impotence due to medication, endometriosis, diabetes, arthritis; almost any medical condition can affect sexual functioning.

The patient with a physical ailment is a whole person with feelings about that disability or disease. Feeling less of a woman or man because of the development of illness may profoundly affect sexual responsiveness and desire. A woman who has had an operation which she regards as mutilating (removal of a breast, or an abdominal scar) may be fairly easy to identify; one whose feeling of damage is concealed (for example, after a cone biopsy or removal of an ovarian cyst) may be more difficult. Patients after any illness or surgery may grieve for their previous good health or completeness and find sexual responsiveness inhibited.

OVERT SEXUAL COMPLAINTS

Because sexual activity is implicitly indicated by the attendance for birth control advice, it is easier for patients to broach the subject with the nurse or doctor (Tunnadine, 1992). Some patients find this easy, others need prompting or require sensitivity to the hesitation or hints. Asking patients routinely, 'Have you any sexual difficulty?' may occasionally be productive but is more likely to elicit a negative response. Such an answer makes it less easy for patients to complain to their advisers at a later date when rapport between them has been better established. Open-ended enquiries such as, 'Any problems?' or 'How are you getting on?' are more likely to enable patients tentatively to sound out doctors and nurses for their response. A reply of, 'No problems really' may need the prompt, 'Does that mean no problems, or a problem that you are not sure whether to mention?' Overtures such as, 'Is it normal for a woman not to have an orgasm?' need to be met by a receptive response. A closed reply like, 'It always takes a while to get the timing right in any relationship' prevents any further exploration of what the complainant means by her enquiry. Although the way the question was put suggests a problem with satisfaction within the sexual act, the real reason may be a lack of desire, a failure of response or a combination of all three. Without an enquiring look or a 'Tell me a bit more', the adviser has no way of understanding the problem being presented. By assuming knowledge, thinking that understanding is present, reassurance or information may be given completely inappropriately. Often, just by telling the doctor or nurse about the problem, patients can see for themselves what causes the difficulty and what they can do about it.

Sometimes patients can make what seems to be an overt complaint but need assistance in order to make the problem clear, not only to the doctor, but also to themselves.

Despite her 20 years, Miss A. looked like a schoolgirl with her white ankle socks and Alice-banded hair. She sat nervously on the edge of her chair, her big eyes gazing trustingly at the doctor. She had just seen the nurse, who had put her through to see the doctor again because she had a problem. 'The nurse said you could sort out this problem I've got,' she confided. The doctor felt wary. What was this problem that had to be handed over to the doctor to be sorted out? 'Tell me about it,' she responded. Miss A. said that she never enjoyed intercourse and her boyfriend was complaining. She stopped. The doctor went, 'Um,' and nodded. 'That's it really.' Miss A. sat back in her chair, problem handed over, ready for instruction. For an instant the doctor was tempted to launch into a lecture or question and answer session on 'How to enjoy intercourse' but recognized the teacher/pupil relationship and restrained herself. 'Tell me a bit more about you and your boyfriend,' she said. 'What do you want to know?' Miss A. countered. The doctor suppressed her irritation, recognizing the 'adolescent child' defiance. She tried to defuse the defence with a smile and said gently, 'It is difficult to know where to begin, isn't it?' and waited. After a moment of bewilderment Miss A. began again. As she progressed through her account she constantly looked for approval that what she was saying was what the doctor wanted. 'Do you want to hear about that?' and 'Perhaps this doesn't matter'. As she told the story it emerged that she lived at home and they had intercourse only occasionally in either her or his parents' house. She was able to discover how nervous she felt about either set of parents knowing what they were doing. She felt like a child in both environments and too young to be sexually active. She felt they should just be cuddling not going 'all the way'. There was a short silence at the end of her account. Then she said, almost as if the doctor was not in the room, 'We're going away on holiday together next month; I think I'll see what it's like then. It might be better away from home.' She came back to the present and said, 'Well, I'd better have some more Pills hadn't I?' excluding the doctor from the previous problems and taking back into privacy her doubts about her sexuality.

This patient had not needed any 'therapy'; she had the answers within herself but needed a skilful listener to enable her to make the transition from 'obedient nonsexual child' to 'independent sexual adult'. By recognizing that the doctor/patient relationship started as teacher/pupil and by refusing to instruct her, the doctor helped Miss A. to take a more adult role, accept the problem as her own, understand the difficulties and see that she could solve it herself. The skill here lies not in what the doctor did but what she restrained herself from doing in response to the initial doctor/patient interaction.

COVERT PRESENTATIONS

Doctors and nurses unskilled in picking up clues about hidden problems may find some contraceptive consultations baffling and frustrating. The patients who can never find a satisfactory method; this Pill made them sick, that one gave them headaches, the coil made them bleed, they had cystitis with the diaphragm, and there is no chance the partner will use a condom. These patients manage to out-manoeuvre and defeat their advisers. Only by understanding that 'nothing is right with contraception' may be a synonym for 'nothing is right with my sexual life' can this be untangled (Rogers, 1989). Sometimes specific complaints with contraception can turn out to have quite different causes.

Miss P. attended a clinic asking for non-allergenic condoms. The nurse enquired why and was told that the patient was allergic to ordinary sheaths. Undetered by the patient's defensive manner, the nurse enquired further and was told that the patient was sore after intercourse. She explained that this might be due to many causes other than allergy and put the patient through to see the doctor. Initially the patient appeared quite angry: 'What was this all about? All I want was the condoms.' The doctor resisted the impulse to give a lecture on the causes of soreness, merely saying that allergy to condoms was really rather rare, and could Miss P. tell her some more about what was wrong? Miss P. then told or how she had started to be sore after intercourse using condoms with her partner about two years previously. She knew it was the condoms because it was all right without, but they usually used condoms because he did not want her to get pregnant. She hastened to explain in some detail that he already had two children by his wife from whom he was separated. The doctor wondered silently why this decision not to get pregnant needed such anxious defence and asked, 'Had you thought about changing to a different method of contraception?' There was a long confused explanation – all about Pills upsetting her and him wanting to look after her and make sure she would not get pregnant – and the doctor did not clearly understand what Miss P. meant. She said, 'It seems to me that you are saying that he needs to be sure that you are not going to get pregnant?' There was a long silence. The doctor looked at Miss P.'s bowed head and eventually reached out and touched her hand saying, 'You have some strong feelings about this?' Miss P. looked away and said in a muffled voice, 'I'm 28 now. I want to get married and leave home and have a family of my own, but he won't get a divorce in case he can't see his children again.' There was another long silence.

'What happened two years ago?' the doctor asked, remembering the length of the history. 'He went back to his wife then but couldn't stand it and left again.' Miss P. compressed her lips and then burst out, 'It isn't fair, I know he would be happy with me but he won't risk getting married again. If only we had a baby, I know it would be all right. He would love a baby, he loves children, he can't bear to be away from his children. If I had his baby it would be all right, he would marry me then,' and she wept, hot, angry, body-jerking tears. When she had sobbed herself to a standstill, work could continue on the real reason for her 'soreness' when condoms were used.

Miss P. had correctly observed the connection between the use of condoms and her soreness; if it had not been for the defensiveness about her explanation of her partner's need for her to avoid pregnancy it might have been accepted at face value and not explored further. How very important it is to pay attention, not just to what is said, but the manner in which it is said.

Patients may present many physical complaints. One attended for a repeat of her contraceptive pill following a termination of pregnancy. She complained of an offensive discharge present since the termination and wondered if she had an infection. Examination revealed a very normal looking vagina and the swabs were all negative. The doctor was then able to discuss with the patient what the termination had meant to her and explore her disgust with herself for what had happened. Another, respectable and dowdy patient, married to a boring, pompous older man, asked to be fitted with a diaphragm and then returned repeatedly asking for an examination and swabs to be taken. The doctor was irritated by the apparently meek approach from the patient and was reluctant to repeat the examination. The patient always managed to manoeuvre the doctor into taking more swabs. When the meaning of this (looking for 'badness') was explored, the patient eventually revealed that she had been a wild teenager and had fantasies that her vagina was the place from which this bad and dangerous person might erupt again. Coming to terms with herself, she was able to recognize that she was deeply unhappy in her relationship with this man whom she had married hoping that he could control the dangerous side of her nature.

Blair described how giving up the oral contraceptive pill may be a signal of emotional fears and other difficulties such as the relationship with the partner (Blair, 1983). She reported on patients who were requesting termination of pregnancy who had taken the Pill and either given up or taken it irregularly. Some of these patients had fears about their femininity and needed to test them out by becoming pregnant. There were adolescents who were having problems in other areas of their lives and complained that they 'could not take' the Pill. They were having battles with authority figures and wished to demonstrate their sexuality and independence in an irresponsible way. Other patients felt under stress and were resentful of having to take contraceptive pills. They were unable to ask for help with their lives without creating a crisis. Finally, a group was identified where the anxieties projected onto the Pill were actually a sign of stress within the partnership. They could be a cover for an actual dislike of intercourse or frigidity, or an expression of problems such as retarded or premature ejaculation. Many of this group had given up the Pill when they needed it most – just as the relationship was disintegrating.

Doctors and nurses should be cautious when faced with a seemingly innocuous request to change the method or type of contraception.

An immediate agreement that this can be done defuses the aggression and determination not to be talked into continuing with what seems to be the cause of difficulties. Then the situation can be further explored to find out what is behind the anxiety.

Mrs J. had her hair combed into an immaculate French pleat at the back and was wearing a smart business suit. She put her briefcase between herself and the doctor. She wanted to be sterilized and come off the Pill. 'That *man* doctor said I was far too young and would change my mind?' She harrangued the doctor about 'men' and 'patronizing doctors' until this woman doctor felt uncomfortable not agreeing with her. The doctor shuffled the notes around and managed to interject, 'Some doctors are like that but Dr M. is usually quite sensitive and understanding.' Mrs J. stopped her complaints and glared at the doctor accusingly. 'Anyway,' the doctor continued, 'tell me about why you would like to be sterilized.' Mrs J. explained that she was 26 had a responsible executive career and did not want any children. She did not want to go on taking contraceptive pills, she always felt nauseous when she restarted each pack and was sure they could not be doing her body chemistry any good. Other methods? They were quite disgusting or barbaric or just unreliable, so she had decided on sterilization. 'What about your partner?' the doctor queried. 'My husband,' she emphasized, 'understands that my career must come first.' There was an expression of contempt on her face. The doctor, attempting to understand the contempt, tried out: 'It sounds to me as if you wish he *would* disagree.' Mrs J. was less strident, 'Oh, he never stands up for himself – he likes a quiet life.' There was a long pause. 'He can't even get an erection half the time now,' she said, looking more vulnerable. 'He offered to have a vasectomy, but I thought it might make the erection problem worse.' With the loss of her defensive hostility, the doctor was able to talk with Mrs J. about her relationship. Her need always to be seen to be in charge at work and how difficult it was to switch off when she was at home. How she wanted him to be assertive (and erect). She did not ask about sterilization again, had a routine check and renewal of the Pill and left, promising to return if things were not improving.

This patient's hostility and need to be in charge had alienated one doctor and provoked him into retaliation. Uncharacteristically, he had told her that he would not do what she wanted; he had met her aggression with an attack by telling her she did not know what she wanted. He was right, but had not understood why, and had used her age as a 'reason' for refusal. The failure to examine what was behind her demand led to more determination on her part to get what she wanted – a release from her difficulties within her relationship which she had inappropriately focussed onto the Pill. The second doctor had recognized the hostility and the need to be in charge and had become, also uncharacteristically, diffident and tentative, while still remaining 'in charge'. Rather than challenging head-on, the doctor tried sneaking in round the back by allowing the patient to explain her reasoning. Only when Mrs J. was able to explain the circumstances behind her demand could she begin to see that what she was doing was illogical. She could then appreciate that her difficulties could not be solved by a change in her method of contraception but only by changes in her relationship with her husband.

Anxiety about a contraceptive method may be a reasonable, logical result of some adverse or misunderstood publicity. Any change in the perceived harm/benefit ratio may cause an inappropriately large shift towards disuse or change. Adverse effects are always more newsworthy than benefits. For example, articles about possible links between oral contraceptives and breast cancer received prominent publicity in all the main newspapers, but other articles showing that a link could not always be shown received little or no mention. The perception of the public who only obtain their information from the media is always slanted towards the dramatic presentation of bad news. So they come to believe that the Pill causes breast cancer, that the intrauterine device gives people infections, that spermicides make babies deformed, that sterilization leads to hysterectomies, and that sheaths are faulty and have holes in them. These misunderstandings need to be understood, not just refuted, otherwise doctors invite the response, 'Well, they would say that, wouldn't they!'

Problems tend to present because of specific triggering factors and often with changes in circumstances. Some patients seem to have difficulty in accepting that they can have enough control over their own lives to choose to use birth control. The woman who staggers from one crisis to another bewailing that 'Everything happens to me' often seems powerless to decide for herself what should happen.

Miss B. originally attended with her partner for a new patient interview. They were an incongruous pair: he was grubby with a marked local accent, wearing torn jeans and with his hair in a pony-tail, while she was a slim, neat girl with a well-educated voice. He did all the talking and was concerned because she was always feeling ill. Some tests were arranged and the doctor was relieved when she reattended by herself. Miss B. ignored the test results and reassurance offered. Her boyfriend had told her to get a coil fitted. She said that after the enquiries at the last consultation (when he had assured the doctor that contraception was not a problem), he had thought about it and decided that as he did not want any children about the place, she had better get fixed up. Suggestions that she might have some opinions or feelings about it were met with a look of incomprehension and after battling for a while – 'I must have a coil today', she kept saying – the doctor gave her some leaflets to read and arranged to see her with her period the following week. At that consultation, she arrived in complete distress, her boyfriend having been picked up in possession of drugs. Decisions were postponed. Next time she was more composed and 'they' had decided she would go back on the Pill, which she had taken 'for several years'. Further enquiry revealed that her boyfriend was on remand and likely to be sent to prison. Naively the doctor enquired why contraception was necessary, only to discover that Miss B. lived in a multi-occupied house and without her boyfriend's presence would be expected to be available to the other men living there. The doctor, sure by now that there were deep underlying problems, probed and listened and encouraged until the girl, relaxed and open, was able to reveal that she had been dominated totally by her authoritarian solicitor father and sexually abused by him until she was 20. She had then met her present boyfriend through her black sheep brother who had rebelled against her father and was into drugs and various criminal activities. She had been thrown out of her home only to join another abusive environment, and had no idea

of how to take control over her own life or sexuality.
She saw herself as available to be used and only considered contraception as a necessary part of this.

This woman's lack of awareness that she had any rights over her
body, her acceptance of the authority of the boyfriend and the urgency
in her need to comply with his instructions about contraception, all
pointed to a deeper disturbance. The irritation felt by the doctor with
this lack of self-determination had to be controlled in the search to
make sense of it all. How much easier it would have been just to
be authoritarian in turn and tell her what she must do!

BEGINNING SEXUAL ACTIVITY

It is common to encounter young girls who are very uncertain about
choosing a method of contraception. They attend and request advice
on methods, but are disinclined to choose one; nothing seems quite
right. Suggestions that they should postpone sexual activity may
be met with verbal agreement, often apparent relief, only for the
doctor to discover later that intercourse is still continuing. They
are encouraged to use a reliable method by their advisers but
seem unable to comprehend the need to use it sensibly, often
missing their contraceptive pills, or complaining that it does not
suit them or that the condom or diaphragm makes them sore.
It is as though by not using contraception they are saying, 'I am not
really active sexually, you see, I'm not even managing to use
contraception. This sexual activity is not my responsibility; the onus
is on my partner to make the running.' They often seem surprised
if a pregnancy occurs as though their sexual activity is divorced from
real life.

Others at this stage in their emotional development are still trying
to assert their individuality and establish themselves as adults in the
eyes of authority (parents and other parental figures such as teachers
and social workers). The irony is that they do so in an irresponsible
way, demonstrating to the parental figures that they cannot be relied
upon to be sensible and adult. For this group, becoming pregnant
is often a subconscious way of proving to the parent that they are
old enough to be treated as an adult, so they forget their Pills and
fail to turn up for their repeat appointments.

Peer group pressure may make some girls attend for contraception when they do not need any. Their regular attendance and acceptance of packets of Pills may hide a hidden desperation that they are not like other girls.

Miss K. was a lovely girl who looked like a model, tastefully made up, a little too thin, but beautifully and elegantly dressed. The doctor felt old, untidy and frumpy. The list of contraceptive consultations was quite long, as she had started and stopped the Pill several times. At the last attendance three months previously she had given a history of being on her period and wishing to restart the Pill as she had a new relationship. A previous doctor had written rather peevishly that she refused to consider using condoms (and underlined *'fifth partner in six years'*. She had been asked to return for a cervical smear as she had not yet had one. The doctor noticed that there was no cervical smear form in the notes and started to look for one to fill in. Miss K. tipped back her head moving her long hair back slightly from covering part of her face and said, 'Oh, didn't you see what nurse has written? I'm on my period this week.' The doctor looked at the record and felt quite unreasonably cross: 'You knew that you were due for a smear; why didn't you come two weeks ago when your appointment . . . ' and just caught herself before the accusation was completed. More gently she changed tack. 'I notice that you've been coming to this clinic for six years and have managed to avoid having a smear all that time. That takes some doing!' The girl shrugged her shoulders and did not look at the doctor, who felt another surge of annoyance. What was going on? The doctor tried again. 'It seems to me that you might find the thought of having a smear rather frightening?' No response except a twitch of the shoulders, turning away and excluding the doctor. She tried again. 'Why do you think you don't want to have a smear?' Miss K. muttered something into her hair. The doctor had to ask her to repeat it. 'I just don't want it done.' The doctor waited but nothing was forthcoming, and she pressed again, feeling frustrated, 'I feel very shut out from what you must be feeling.'

Suddenly the memory of the 'fifth partner in six years' flashed into the doctor's mind. Tentatively she continued, 'I noticed in your records that you have changed partners several times. Do you find it difficult to let them into how you are feeling as well?' The girl muttered again and the doctor just caught, 'One of the doctors said I didn't need a smear if I wasn't doing it.' 'Wasn't doing what?' asked the doctor stupidly, and then realized what Miss K. had said. 'Oh, you mean that you're not having intercourse. Why do you keep coming for the Pill, then?' (Oh dear, thought the doctor, I'm really making a mess of this.) The girl lifted her head enough to give the doctor a glimpse of dark brown eyes and dilated pupils. 'Tricia brings me down with her every time I start going out with a new man. She's worried that I'll get pregnant like she did, but there's no chance of that!' and she laughed harshly. The doctor felt very intrusive and clumsy. 'Do you want to tell me about it?' There was a long pause and then Miss K. gave a great shuddering sigh. 'I don't think I can,' she whispered. There was another pause. 'Could I see you again next time I come?' she said and then, with a great effort, 'You won't make me have one of those things?' and gestured at the couch. 'Not until you're ready,' promised the doctor, feeling very protective, and made special arrangements to see Miss K. herself in two weeks.

Here was a girl pretending to her friend and to the clinic that she was sexually active. She changed her partners frequently, perhaps because they became too pressing for intimacy, or because, like the doctor, they were made to feel clumsy and intrusive. Her lack of sexual activity was not through choice and her avoidance of contact with the genital area was clearly shown by her manoeuvres to avoid her cervical smear. Even confessing to the doctor that she was not having intercourse was preferable to being examined. She provoked in the doctor a strong wish to protect her from intrusion and assault. The doctor would need to guard against continuing to collude with Miss K.'s need to be protected. Otherwise no progress in the examination (both of the psychological reasons for the defensiveness and of the physical body) would be made.

RELATIONSHIP PROBLEMS

Complaints that the method of contraception is affecting sexual performance or desire, especially if frequently presented, can indicate a problem within the relationship which the patient does not wish to face. The anxieties are focused on the method of contraception; the fantasy is that, if only this could be made all right, so would the relationship. Doctors are often aware that underlying relationship problems may be behind the request for sterilization or vasectomy (or to stop contraception to have a baby to 'mend' the marriage), but sometimes forget that such difficulties may be behind an otherwise reasonable-sounding request.

> Miss L. was an attractive 18-year-old. She had come to have a coil fitted. The doctor asked why she wanted to change her method. She stuck her jaw forward and said that she had been on the Pill for two years and had gone off sex. She was sure it was the Pill and wanted a coil instead. She looked away from the doctor, not wanting any more discussion (or perhaps to avoid persuasion that this was not the right choice). The doctor waited but no more was forthcoming. 'Tell me a bit more about when you first noticed you were going off sex,' she prompted. With lots of 'ums' and encouraging nods from the doctor, Miss L. hesitantly told her story. She had known her boyfriend since she was 15, and she thought it was time that they got engaged but he did not want to commit himself. As she told the doctor about keeping her evenings free for him and how he then went out with his mates instead, her anger became evident. The doctor picked this up and used it to show her how dissatisfied she was. As they talked, Miss L. gradually realized that she could not change her young man's behaviour and became thoughtful. She decided to postpone having a coil fitted. The next time she was seen, for an unrelated problem, the doctor noticed that

she must have run out of Pills and asked her about it. Miss L. explained that she had stopped taking the Pill. 'We had a big bust up. I started playing badminton with a girl from work and was out one night when he wanted to see me. I told him he didn't own me and some other home truths about how selfish he was – he didn't like it at all and I haven't seen him for weeks now. Good riddance, is what I say!' and she flashed a smile as she went out.

This patient presented a sexual problem which she envisaged as being due to the Pill. She had difficulty in reconciling her fantasy script of love, engagement and marriage to her childhood sweetheart, with the reality of a relationship with a selfish and immature youth. She needed the opportunity to expose the reality and to have her anger acknowledged as a reasonable response to it. Although many people had told her previously that this boy was not husband material, she had hidden the knowledge behind the defence of a sexual problem due to her method of contraception. The doctor, by recognizing the defensiveness and refusing to take the problem at face value, had enabled her to look behind the defences at the real problem.

TROUBLE WITH BABIES

Another common time for a patient to present with difficulties about sexuality or contraception is when a pregnancy, either her own or another's, has occurred; or after delivery.

A woman may present wanting to change from her secure Pill or injection. She may say she is getting older and has been on this method a long time; it must be time for a change. Further exploration may expose anxieties about her fertility with increasing age or that her friends have been having babies.

Intellectually she may not want to get pregnant – it may be the wrong time financially or for her career – but she no longer feels easy with absolute control over her fertility and she wants to take a risk. In that way she does not have to decide logically and sensibly that she wants a baby: it just happens by chance. Sometimes just demonstrating that she is fertile is enough. Perversely to her medical attendants, once pregnant she may want a termination (see Chapter 4). Or she may leap at the opportunity to abandon what was, for her, an imposed choice of job over motherhood.

Other patients have difficulty seeing themselves as sexual once they become parents. They cannot imagine their own parents behaving sexually (although intellectually they know they must have done so), and have problems re-establishing sexual activity for pleasure after delivery. The emotional demands a new baby makes on the mother, and the intense bonding that occurs, the physical tiredness, the hormonal changes and even depression, all conspire to exclude the husband and diminish the wife's desire for closeness with him. Some mothers may even say they do not need birth control, and not use it or refuse intercourse until they want to become pregnant again. For some, motherhood is the only role in which they feel fulfilled.

Fear of pregnancy may inhibit sexual responsiveness. Patients who feel that a baby would be a disaster, or have had previous failure of their contraceptive method may need frequent reassurance about the method. They may reattend with complaints that the withdrawal bleed is too short or too long, or that they felt sick and were not sure that they had absorbed the Pill, or that the tenderness of the breasts must mean that they are pregnant despite the regular bleeding. The amenorrhoea following use of injectables may require frequent pregnancy tests, or there may be repeated requests for emergency contraception because of anxieties about whether the condom was used correctly. A previous unfortunate experience (a stillbirth, neonatal death, or an eventful pregnancy or delivery) may make the woman fearful of another disaster. Another reason for apprehension may be the fear of disapproval of sexual activity which would become evident to the world outside if the woman becomes pregnant. Attendance for contraception can be hidden; a pregnant abdomen much less so. The responsibility for the sexual activity becomes vested in the doctor: if pregnancy occurs it is the doctor's failure, not the patient's sexuality which has caused it.

AM I TOO OLD FOR SEX?

Diffidence about asking for contraception or with continuing it may occur as part of a difficulty in accepting the sexual activity of 'older' women. One woman said she hated attending the family planning clinic because it was 'full of young girls who look at you as if you were a dirty old woman'. A family planning nurse said at a conference on the needs of young people that the over-40s could do with separate clinics to protect them from embarrassment as well. The frequency of marital break-up means that many women are faced with a sudden upsurge in their sexual activity and a need for excellent contraception within a new partnership after many years of needing little or no contraception, the partner having had a vasectomy, or from lack of intercourse. One older woman, after several years of absence from the family planning clinic, brought to the clinic doctor the photograph of her new partner, as well as sharing her intense excitement in this new sexual relationship. She could not share it with anyone else, as she felt they would think her disgusting and lustful. The request for contraception needs to be considered together with the social behaviour making it necessary. There is plenty of potential for preventive work in every consultation. A calm acceptance of sexual activity at any age helps to make patients feel more comfortable about discussing their contraceptive and sexual needs.

FURTHER TREATMENT OR REFERRAL?

It is not always possible to identify and deal with problems as they arise in the consultation although such immediate management would be ideal. The constraints of time are inevitable: the average appointment in general practice is seven to ten minutes in length, and in a clinic the pressure from the other staff to keep up with the flow of patients may be expressed openly by interruptions or reminders of the queue of other patients waiting to be seen. Most simple, straightforward problems are best dealt with at the time that they are discovered or presented, before they are established into a malfunctioning system of behaviour. Others will need more time and effort, or require referral.

Patients also provide constraints. Just because a problem is revealed does not necesarily mean that the patient wishes to do some work on it. It may not be the right time for the patient to look at the difficulty exposed, perhaps unwittingly. A patient who revealed for the first time at the age of 38 years, that she had been sexually abused as a child, because of something that had been picked up by the doctor during a routine cervical smear, did not wish to take up the doctor's offer of another appointment or referral to discuss it further. She felt it was better left buried (as it had been for many years), despite her difficulty in responding sexually to her husband.

Patients may want to have time to come to terms with what has been exposed before discussing it further or deciding to do nothing. Sometimes patients wish to keep their sexual problems, or indeed their contraceptive needs, separate from the management of their illnesses and ask to be referred elsewhere. There may be practical problems for a GP when the partner of a patient needs to be seen but is not registered. A woman can be registered for 'contraception only' services, but this often is not available where the male partner needs to be seen, and referral may be necessary.

Then there are the constraints provided by the doctor. The doctor may feel unable to give help because of an awareness of lack of aptitude or skill. Or doctors may find that personal feelings are interfering with the proper objective management of the problems, particularly if similar problems have been experienced personally or to someone emotionally close to them. For example, it may be too distressing to cope with a patient complaining of lack of libido after a miscarriage of a wanted baby if the doctor or the doctor's wife has recently suffered the same misfortune. It may be impossible to deal with a patient giving a history of sexual abuse if the doctor finds that personal memories and distress are re-awakened. Sometimes social contacts may also make it necessary for doctors to distance themselves from the problem. It is not a good idea, for instance, to take on one's colleagues for therapy, however much they may want to keep it 'in the family'. Friends and acquaintances are not well served by agreement to help them informally – a referral to a colleague where a proper patient/therapist relationship can maintain professional standards is in everybody's best interest.

Sensitive, caring doctors, who pick up the clues of distress from their patients, are often tempted to carry too great a burden. Patients bring their problems to doctors but ultimately have to sort them out themselves. They can be helped to examine the difficulties, but doctors cannot do the work for them. The patient may easily develop a dependent parent/child relationship with the doctor and fail to take on the responsibility for change. A tired doctor, burnt out from the demands made by dependent patients, is unable to see clearly the processes occurring between the patient and the doctor. Full atttention is needed to identify the interactions which explain how and why the patient presented at that particular time, to recognize the hidden needs behind the spoken complaints, and to use the feelings arising during the consultation to help the patient to understand the nature of the problems.

Training to improve skills in this work should be sought by anyone who is encountering many patients with sexual difficulties. Information about training is available from the Institute of Psychosexual Medicine (see p. XIV). Perhaps those who work in family planning and are not seeing patients with sexual problems should examine their consultation skills (see Chapter 13) to discover what prevents patients revealing their difficulties. The aim of basic training should be to learn to make a diagnosis in sexually related problems, know which can be treated in the setting in which they present and in the time available, and which patients should be referred elsewhere. Doctors who want, and are suitable, to make this a field of special interest should go on to more specialized further training and may be able, then, to treat more complex and time-consuming problems in separate sessions outside their normal working environment.

Sometimes referral represents a flight from the complaints presented by the patient; at other times it may be a necessity because of over-involvement with the patient's difficulties or emotions.

Mrs S. was a favourite with the doctor. She was a bubbly woman, confident and attractive, who had worked hard to educate herself and had achieved an Open University degree and a post as a legal executive after an upbringing in a working class family. She rarely consulted except for contraception and the doctor felt her husband, a professional man whom the doctor knew socially was a lucky man to have snapped up such a peach. The doctor was disappointed when Mrs S. failed to attend for a contraceptive consultation and sent in a request for a prescription to tide her over until she could make another appointment. When she next attended, she looked rather strained and said she was thinking of changing from the oral contraceptive she had been on for some time. Could she have some leaflets to think about what would be the best for her? The doctor enquired why she wanted to change from a method that had suited her for several years. She said, rather distantly that she was not so sure that it had been suiting her but declined to expand on her statement, saying only that she would return when she had made up her mind what to do. The doctor felt excluded and baffled.

He was pleased when she returned and told him that she did not know what to do. He had the bright idea that perhaps she wanted a pregnancy (she was now 34 years old) and wanted a less certain method so that she could become pregnant by accident rather than making a definite decision about a family. She shot him down. There was no question of her wanting a child. Her husband, she reminded him, had three rising teenagers by his previous wife, quite enough to cope with. And for herself, she had never wanted children, and was pleased to find a partner who would not put any pressure on her in that direction. The Pill was so convenient and reliable, all the other methods seemed so hit and miss. What did he think her chances of being sterilized were? Perhaps, she rushed him onwards, she could have it done privately. The doctor struggled to regain the initiative. *Why* did she want to stop the Pill? She was healthy with no risk factors and could continue on for several years yet if she wanted. He waited and rather wished he had not confronted her, as the silence became very uncomfortable. Just as he was thinking perhaps he should just agree to refer her for sterilization, she seemed to make up her mind to confide in him. She told him that she had never had any satisfaction making love with her husband. Mr S. thought that she did not reach orgasm because she was on the Pill, but, blushing, she was able to tell the doctor that she had been orgasmic with other partners before her husband, and had been on the Pill then. She told him that she had not minded at first, she had thought it was just that he was so ardent and passionate that he came so quickly and could not hold back. She had thought that as their relationship became more mature and less urgent he would slow down, but he always came as soon as he was inside her, and sometimes before.

The doctor was in a quandary. He wanted to help her; wanted to ask her to bring her husband to see him, but felt alarmed by his feelings of anger towards the husband, and that he himself could do better given half a chance. To give himself time to think, he said he would make some enquiries about sources of help for them and arranged to see her again, leaving her contraception, by mutual agreement, unchanged.

He presented the consultation to his training seminar, expecting condemnation for his personal feelings, and hoping to understand his confusion by discussion with members of the group. The seminar appreciated his dilemma. There was agreement that he had to maintain his professional relationship with Mrs S. and concentrate on his role as a doctor and not as a rival to her husband. There was no evidence that the husband thought he had a problem, and he would not be likely to co-operate if dragged along 'for treatment' by his wife. If the wife wanted help to sort out her complaint (that her husband had premature ejaculation), he should refer her. She could then negotiate with her husband whether he was willing to participate in therapy, in order to improve her sexual satisfaction. The doctor expressed his relief; he had been torn between his personal feelings that here was a dangerous situation, and his professional pride.

Although this doctor had a special interest in psychosexual therapy and some skill in this field, his personal feelings made therapy with this woman, or her husband, a potential minefield. The professional pride of this doctor nearly led him to embark on a dangerous offer of therapy. He could recognize that, because of his training, he had been able to stick with the real problem – that the woman wanted to change her method of contraception without the existence of a logical acceptable reason. He knew from his previous experience with similar encounters that an emotional reason was likely. He had several bright ideas: she might feel she was too old to be continuing on the combined oral contraceptive, or that she might want a less reliable method in order to risk pregnancy without taking a definite decision to start a family. The failure of these ideas to strike a chord with the patient reminded the doctor that each patient is unique and that experience gained from other patients is of no help in understanding what is happening with this particular patient. Only when he waited, in ignorance, for her to tell him what the problem was for her, did he discover the underlying difficulty. He knew, too, that if the husband had come to him with the problem of premature ejaculation, he might have been able to help him discover why it happened. Perhaps his first wife had taken too much from him and he wanted subconsciously to retain the sexual pleasure for himself; perhaps he had always had this pattern and could not see any difficulty, or any of the myriad other reasons why it occurs. Then he could perhaps help him to make the necessary changes to ovecome the precipitate ejaculation. The doctor's difficulty was his nonprofessional partisan feelings, which made referral elsewhere a preferable option. He would have to propose this to Mrs S. without making her feel rejected.

Referral should take place after mutual agreement between the patient (who is complaining) and the doctor. The purpose is to obtain a specialist opinion, or investigations or treatment not available from the referring doctor. Reluctance or even resistance will be encountered if the patient has been sent by another person, such as the partner, for treatment, when they do not perceive that they have a problem (as with Mr S.). It might be possible to suggest to a partner that the patient complaining will need the assistance of that partner in the therapy, thus engaging their interest at the outset.

However, if the doctor insists on referring both partners when only one is complaining, there may be serious difficulties for the therapist to whom the couple are referred. Both partners need to accept an adult and responsible role during therapy. The therapist offers interpretation and suggestions about changes, but it is up to the individuals to make use of them. More often, a therapist, whether using cognitive therapy, behavioural techniques or psychotherapeutic interpretations, will empathize with the person who seeks help for the problem. A partner who has not acknowledged that he or she has a problem is much harder to engage in therapy, and may opt out by not attending either physically or mentally, or even undermining therapeutic endeavours in a subtle fashion.

Before referral it is important for patients to know and to be able to have some say in the sort of therapist that they would like to see. It is pointless referring a man with impotence to a marital therapist if he wants to see a urologist for physical investigations. The referring doctor needs to be aware of the specific skills which are available, and to keep a balance between the physical and emotional needs of the patient, so that the whole patient can be treated.

Referral may be to a counsellor who is trained to work either with the individual or the couple (or sometimes the family). It is essential that the counsellor is known to be comfortable with sexual issues and to be able to make people comfortable talking about them in private. Counsellors who have had training in sexual therapy will be able to discuss the basic facts about normal sexual functioning, and draw out from the patient or couple ideas about how they might modify their sexual activity, or alter their interaction to improve the difficulties. Counsellors are often particularly helpful where there are communication difficulties between a couple. Counsellors should have recognized training, such as a BA in counselling studies, social work, psychological or psychiatric training, and have continuing supervision and a code of ethics. There are many unqualified counsellors, who may well do a good job, but may equally well project their own prejudices or difficulties onto their clients. A psychiatric social worker or community psychiatric nurse may have special skills in this area, but is more likely to be of help where other disturbances are affecting sexual functioning as well: for example, in a hypomanic patient who is exhibiting inappropriate sexual behaviour, or a depressed individual with loss of libido.

Marital therapists, or couple therapists, work with the couple on the relationship between them. Referral for marital therapy will be more effective when there is agreement between the couple that changes in the relationship are required. Specific training in sexual difficulties is taken by selected therapists who work for Relate Marriage Guidance, or facilities may be available within a psychiatric department. The objective is to establish an emotionally secure relationship which permits normal sexual responses to occur and be enjoyed. The main emphasis is on the nature of the sexual inter-action and away from the specific sexual response. It is essential for this therapy that both of the couple are willing to work at the goals set by the therapist. Based on Masters and Johnson's work (1970), the couple are asked to carry out certain sexual homework assignments while keeping within limits such as the exclusion of genital touching or intercourse in the initial stages. The reaction of the couple to these assignments is then used to examine the interaction between them and to reveal some of the underlying problems. Modern modifications to the original Masters and Johnson techniques include a much more flexible approach using psychotherapeutic methods to identify and reduce the obstacles to the behavioural assignments

(Bancroft 1989). Some therapists work as co-therapists, each working with one of a couple and conferring on how best to proceed together. Others work alone treating a couple and their relationship.

Individual therapy may be available from doctors accredited as members of the Institute of Psychosexual Medicine. The aim of this psychosomatic approach is to promote understanding of the unique nature of each doctor/patient interaction and the help it gives in unravelling the patient's sexual problems. Patients who are referred should be clear that they are to see a doctor who will examine not just their sexual problem but also their physical body.

This psychosomatic approach is a narrow focus on the sexual problems in an otherwise mentally healthy patient. It is particularly suitable for patients where only one of a couple owns the problem, or where there are two complaining patients within a couple who need to be seen separately, or where somatic complaints accompany the emotional difficulties.

Patients who are more globally disturbed with a neurotic or psychotic illness, in which sexual dysfunction is only one of many symptoms, are more appropriately referred to a psychiatrist or psychotherapist for help.

Specific investigations or treatment may be required from other specialists. For example, a gynaecologist may be asked for relief of the dyspareunia caused by endometriosis, or for help with physical problems affecting sexual function (about which the patient will also have feelings). The assistance of an urologist, neurologist or other specialist may be required for other sophisticated physical investigations or treatments, while the primary care physician keeps a close eye on the psychological aspects. The intricate links between feelings and physical symptoms and signs must not be neglected.

CONCLUSION

Contraceptive consultations are favoured occasions for revealing overt or covert sexual problems. By attending for advice on birth control, patients are already revealing that part of them that is sexual, and the subject of difficulties with their sexual life can be broached with less difficulty (it is never easy). Doctors and nurses concerned with giving contraceptive advice should be comfortable discussing sexual matters. They need to be skilful in their ability to receive and manage their patients' confidences and to recognize when and how to refer those they are unable to help.

REFERENCES

Bancroft, J. (1989) Couple therapy, in *Human Sexuality and its Problems*, 2nd edn, Churchill Livingstone, London, p. 467.

Blair, M. (1983) Emotional significance of anxieties about the Pill, in *Practice of Psychosexual Medicine* (ed. K. Draper), J. Libbey, London.

Herzberg, B., Draper, K., Johnson, A. *et al.* (1971) Oral contraceptives, depression and libido. *British Medical Journal*, 3(773), 495–50.

Masters, W.H. and Johnson, V.E. (1970) *Human Sexual Inadequacy*, Churchill Livingstone, London.

Rogers, J. (1989) Presentation of a psychosexual problem, in *Introduction to Psychosexual Medicine* (ed. R. Skrine), Chapman & Hall, London.

Tunnadine, P. (1992) *Insights into Troubled Sexuality*, Chapman & Hall, London.

13

Analysis of the family planning consultation

Sam Rowlands

SUMMARY

- Models of consultation
- The time factor
- Rapport
- Patient's agenda
- Doctor's agenda
- Negotiating a plan
- Discussing follow-up
- Self-monitoring
- Satisfaction

Medical consultations, particularly in general practice, are complicated interpersonal transactions. The family planning consultation is fundamentally no different from other consultations. Along with many other problems which are presented to doctors whose content is not to do with illness, a different approach is needed from that which many doctors were taught at medical school. In addition, the content of family planning consultations is sensitive and delicate, as has been demonstrated in Chapter 12. Both parties need to be comfortable talking about sex for the consultation to succeed. As McEwan (1982) has put it, 'More successful consulting techniques in family planning involve providing the scientific or biomedical knowledge about methods, against a background of nondirective counselling in relation to the social and practical elements of applying the advice to everyday life in sexual relationships.'

One of the ways of helping doctors and other health care workers to provide better contraceptive services is to study what happens in the consultation. Such study can help the doctor to acquire the skill of becoming entangled with the patient's problem and then stepping back and thinking about what is happening. In this chapter mainly the process of the consultation is considered; outcomes of consultations are less well researched and hopefully more can be included in future editions of this book.

MODELS OF THE CONSULTATION

Over the last two decades, doctors and psychologists have attempted to construct models of the consultation which give insight into the complex interactions between doctors and patients.[1] Even earlier, methods of effective counselling had been developed which greatly enhanced communication within a consultation.

The first attempt to categorize consultations grew out of good counselling practice and concerned the different types of intervention doctors could make (Heron, 1975). Interventions were broadly grouped as either authoritarian or facilitative, the former representing the more traditional medical behaviour and the latter being more patient-centred. Authoritarian interventions comprised prescriptive ('the IUCD is a good method for you'), informative and confronting categories. Facilitative interventions were grouped into: (1) cathartic, that is, allowing release of emotion; (2) catalytic, encouraging the client in his train of thought ('Go on', 'Hmm' and so on from the doctor); or (3) supportive ('I understand' or a nonverbal nod of the head).

The consultation was first broken down into phases in work done in Manchester, where nearly 2000 audiotaped consultations

---

[1]Throughout the book the word 'patient' rather than 'client' is used as there is a different relationship with professionals who conduct physical examinations. However, illness-oriented thinking is not appropriate for healthy individuals coming for contraceptive care.

1. The doctor establishes a relationship with the patient.
2. The doctor either attempts to discover or actually discovers the reason for the patient's attendance.
3. The doctor conducts a verbal or a physical examination or both.
4. The doctor, or the doctor and the patient, or the patient (in that order of probability) consider the condition.
5. The doctor, and occasionally the patient, details treatment or further investigation.
6. The consultation is terminated, usually by the doctor.

Figure 13.1. The Byrne and Long consultation model (1976).

were analysed (Byrne and Long, 1976). Six phases were defined which appeared frequently to follow each other in sequence, but the emphasis was still very much on the doctor (Figure 13.1).

Next the consultation was viewed from the angle of maximizing the potential of each consultation, and not just dealing with the presenting problem and getting the patient out through the door (Stott and Davis, 1979). This important work described how other key elements of care, such as the management of continuing problems and opportunistic health promotion, could be raised when appropriate. However, it did not help doctors to understand where they were in the progress through a consultation.

One of the classic texts has been that of Pendleton, Schofield, Tate *et al.* (1984), which for the first time emphasized the importance of taking into account the patient's ideas, concerns and expectations and involving the patient in the process of understanding the problem and working out solutions (Figure 13.2). Without wishing in any way to undermine the achievement of this work, doctors may find their model rather theoretical and difficult to hold in mind while consulting.

Two further workers have refined the comprehensive Oxford model and, arguably, made it more accessible and immediate. Neighbour (1987) condensed the seven tasks of the consultation into five (Figure 13.3). His innovative book raised for the first time the intuitive element in the way a consultation is conducted. His illustrations from analysis of videotapes are delightful and can fundamentally change one's approach to consulting.

1. To define the reasons for the patient's attendance, including:
   (a) the nature and history of the problem;
   (b) their aetiology;
   (c) the patient's ideas, concerns and expectations;
   (d) the effects of the problems.
2. To consider other problems:
   (a) continuing problems;
   (b) at-risk factors.
3. To choose with the patient an appropriate action for each problem.
4. To achieve a shared understanding of the problems with the patient.
5. To involve the patient in the management and encourage him or her to accept appropriate responsibility.
6. To use time and resources appropriately.
7. To establish or maintain a relationship with the patient which helps to achieve the other tasks.

Figure 13.2 Consultation model conceived by Pendleton, Schofield, Tate and Havelock (1984).

1. Connecting
2. Summarizing
3. Handing over
4. Safety-netting
5. Housekeeping

Figure 13.3 Neighbour's consultation model (1987).

Finally, Middleton (1989) produced the most recent paper which is simplicity itself. Communication skills are used to reconcile the respective agendas of both doctor and patient into a jointly negotiated plan.

Distilling what this author considers to be the best of these various models, a scheme has been made which is helpful for consultations which have minimal illness content and can be used by the doctor during a consultation (Figure 13.4). The headings in this chapter refer back to this scheme.

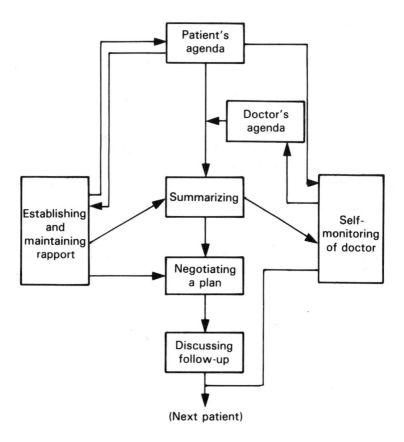

Figure 13.4 Scheme of the family planning consultation.

THE TIME FACTOR

Many doctors fear that adopting the counselling mode will encourage patients to waffle on indefinitely and they will never get home. This fear appears to be misplaced. Considering the importance of ascertaining the reason for the consultation, it is vital to give the patient a fair hearing. Wilkinson (1989) found that three-quarters of general practice patients had finished speaking within one minute and 98% had finished within two minutes.

The other aspect of time and the consultation is that it may take place over long periods as a succession of brief contacts. Analysis of one particular contact might reveal the absence of several critical phases. For example, negotiating a plan might well be omitted in subsequent contacts, once it has been agreed, if a contact is following up that particular problem only.

RAPPORT

It has been shown that positioning chairs in the consulting room so that the doctor and patient face each other across the corner of the desk encourages more verbal interaction than when doctor and patient are on opposite sides of the desk (Pietroni, 1976). Also, it has been estimated that two-thirds of the communication which goes on in a two-person conversation is nonverbal and only one-third verbal.

The beginning of the consultation has proved to be of great interest and of vital importance. Clearly, to get off on the wrong footing may ruin the whole consultation. Neighbour (1987) has analysed this phase in considerable detail. 'Curtain raisers' are little throw-away lines such as, 'You'll be getting fed up with me' which may be missed as the patient enters. The consultation has begun at this stage and interventions from now on can disturb the flow of the consultation. Lines such as 'You *are* busy today, doctor' (really meaning 'you have kept me waiting 40 minutes') may even provoke some anger in the doctor if pressure of work that day is beyond his or her control.

Establishing rapport is to do with making the patient feel at ease. Ascertaining the name the patient likes to be called is useful; it may well be different from the names given at registration. 'Matching' is a technique which may be needed early on to get in touch with the patient; for example, adopting the patient's tone of voice or posture can be a powerful signal that one is adjusting to their wavelength. A patient's diffidence is reduced by these means and worries are thus less likely to be held back.

Does it matter what sort of clothes the doctor wears? Instinctively, one would say that ordinary dress would be more welcoming than white coats. The fact is that GPs tend to wear ordinary clothes in their surgeries and clinic and hospital doctors white coats, and the public are used to this. In one study about clothes in family planning consultations (Stewart and Woodhouse, 1987), the majority of patients in a community clinic setting thought that the doctors should wear white coats. This view extended throughout all age groups, although the majority was not quite so large among the under-20s.

Once rapport has been established, the consultation can proceed more effectively because the doctor/patient relationship is in harmony (Freeling and Harris, 1984). When doctor and patient get to know and trust each other, the first phase of the consultation may become redundant. However, as with all relationships, rapport may have its ups and downs and work may be needed to rebuild rapport from time to time.

PATIENT'S AGENDA

It is important that the patient's agenda always comes before the doctor's agenda. The patient's agenda may be overt or covert (the hidden agenda). The agenda may include that of the partner, whether present or absent at the particular consultation. Family planners encourage patients to bring their partners with them to a consultation. Seeing a couple together may be beneficial so that the method chosen can be one that suits both partners.

Neighbour calls the line which the patient has been rehearsing in the waiting room the 'opening gambit' (1987). The patient may well have more than one of these at the ready. Perhaps a 'respectable' line such as, 'The Pill is giving me these awful headaches, doctor', and a line about her fundamental problem such as, 'My husband is unemployed and has lost all interest in sex', which could be used if the time is felt to be ripe. The respectable line is far more likely to be used with its lower risk, if the doctor does not make good eye contact initially or if he pre-empts the patient's offering by asking a question.

Examples of situations alerting the doctor to a hidden agenda are given by Freeling and Harris (1984). Nonverbal cues may be obtained from the patient's gestures, posture and dress, reflecting an emotional state she or he does not mention. Or the patient's opening gambit may be a general question rather than a statement about the problem. If the doctor suspects a hidden agenda is present, he may want to prompt the patient gently: 'Is there something else you wanted to tell me?' Otherwise it may come out as a throw-away line as the patient is leaving – the 'by the way' syndrome.

Janice, a 26-year-old insulin-dependent diabetic came in to see her GP whom she had known for four years. She was requesting lancets for blood glucose monitoring. On receipt of the prescription she asked if it was possible for her to be referred to a clinic where sexual problems could be discussed. When asked what the problem was she hastily stressed it was *her* problem, not her husband's, and that she had a block when making love.

She then went on to disclose to the GP (having done so two weeks earlier to her husband) the sexual abuse she suffered as a child. She described how her dark secret had recently become unblocked from the recesses of her mind and kept coming to the fore. She was having flashbacks to her abuse and she would freeze and be unable to respond.

After she had talked further to the doctor, she mentioned how she had been tempted to make the disclosure the previous year when being counselled by him about sterilization, but felt she could not inflict this on her husband who was present. She had also contemplated disclosure at other appointments but had either been prevented by a very unpleasant lump in the throat or by being inhibited by the presence of her young children. Although distressed she said she felt considerably unburdened after the disclosure. The GP congratulated her on her courage in talking to him that day. After she had gone out he looked at the number of contacts they had had while she was holding onto her secret. He had personally seen her with an appointment for herself seven times and had visited her at home twice after the birth of one of her children. It had taken nine contacts for trust to develop and the time to be ripe for the disclosure.

Although the doctor and the patient had developed rapport early on in their relationship, a much deeper trust had developed over the years. Nevertheless, Janice could not launch straight into her fundamental agenda item. She brought with her an 'entry-ticket' to the consulting room (requests for lancets) and then proceeded to introduce the hidden agenda with a general question about another problem which she clearly realized was only secondary to the main item. This case illustrates that success often occurs after a series of contacts which make up the overall consultation.

What is the first thing one tends to say to patients? Doctors all have stock phrases such as, 'What can I do for you?' It may be salutary to think about how one intervenes and what effect this may have on the consultation. One can be ultra-specific, perhaps referring back to an earlier problem such as, 'Are you still spotting in the first week of the packet?' which makes assumptions and sets an agenda for the patient based on the doctor's concerns. Welcoming phrases such as, 'Hello, Christine. Come in and sit down' may be preferable. At least one is not asking a question. If one really wants to keep the agenda wide open this author has found 'Yes . . .' to be useful, or even total silence with an expectant look and firm eye contact. The latter example is obviously not appropriate for someone you have never met before. The temptation to use social chit-chat to break the ice: 'Have you had a busy day at work?' should be resisted as it may block the patient's opening gambit. However, listening in stony silence for minimal cues when the patient wants a blood pressure check, a repeat prescription and to dash off to prepare something to eat can be felt as threatening and is a waste of the doctor's and the patient's time.

What about looking at the notes? It is conventional good practice for doctors to try to be well-briefed about the patient sitting before them. Could perhaps this process prevent one from seeing this person with a fresh eye and encourage one to prejudge the person's character, or focus in on previous events which are not on the patient's agenda that particular day? It is tempting to make assumptions about the patient's agenda particularly at a follow-up consultation brought about at the doctor's request.

While the patient is talking, one begins to get a feel about the patient. One may hear snippets about their partner, the family or the workplace and begin to understand their feelings about sex and contraception. Family intentions are very important and relevant to the discussion of different methods. Listening carefully may reveal the sort of conflicts mentioned earlier in this book.

A common practice in family planning clinics is for patients to see the nurse for history-taking and then go in to see the doctor. While fully acknowledging that many patients develop rapport with nurses better than with doctors, this split type of consultation can have disadvantages. Highly trained nurses can run their own consultations independently (the so-called delegation session) unless a medical problem arises or an IUD insertion is required.

Balint (1964) emphasized that if doctors ask questions in the manner of medical history-taking, they will always get answers – but hardly anything more. The main skill in *receiving* the patient's agenda is careful listening. This is not a passive activity – all sorts of ideas, paradoxes and questions may come into the doctor's mind as well as being able to notice verbal cues such as what the patient omits to say or speech idiom and nonverbal cues such as facial expression or posture. Skilled doctors can ask questions which are relevant to what the patient is talking about which, although interruptions, may be facilitative and may maintain or even encourage the flow of the consultation,

One important cue which Neighbour (1987) describes and had entirely passed this author by is the 'internal search'. While a patient is intent on remembering or imagining something important, the body becomes relatively still and the eyes defocused and fixed in position. While attention is directed inwards, thoughts and memories begin to associate in the imagination. Sometimes an internal search follows a question the doctor has asked and the patient may finish up with a new insight into the problem. It is important not to interrupt anyone during an internal search.

The quality of empathy is required of the doctor. Freeling and Harris (1984) define empathy as putting oneself imaginitively into someone else's position and experiencing the feelings which doing so arouses. These feelings will be returned to under the heading of 'Self-monitoring' below.

DOCTOR'S AGENDA

The doctor's agenda may be either relevant or irrelevant to the patient. Clearly the doctor may have personal problems which get in the way; there may be preconceived ideas about a particular patient or about certain types of patient (sometimes triggered by appearance or dress). The doctor may have a stereotype of the patient's partner which is unhelpful: assumptions may be made about age, numbers of partners, sexual orientation or acceptable sexual activities. The doctor may find it difficult to view a patient he known from birth as a sexual adult and so tend to dominate the consultation in an authoritarian style.

If the doctor's beliefs and values intrude into the consultation, concern and empathy may suffer. If the doctor does not believe in abortion, then referral should be organized to a colleague when a termination is requested. If the doctor is uncomfortable talking about how to put on condoms, different positions for lovemaking, masturbation, or does not believe sex should be fun, then the patient will sense this and not feel encouraged to continue talking about the problem.

Patients may have continuing problems of which the doctor is aware, and which may or may not be relevant to refer to in a particular consultation. An example would be a relationship difficulty which might itself need attention in its own right or because of its direct bearing on the presenting problem, for instance a request for a change of method of contraception.

Risk factors can be assessed, in particular noting any new ones since the last attendance. Opportunistic health promotion is the other item which comes from the Stott and Davis model (1979). This may be irrelevant on some occasions, for example, a request for emergency contraception. The term includes screening (cervical cytology, rubella immune status and blood pressure checks for those using non-hormonal methods) and positive health promotion (help with giving up smoking, dietary advice, suggestions for improving relationships with the patient's partner and raising the question of safer sex and reducing risk of sexually transmitted diseases, including HIV infection).

Doctors will need to follow their routine medical procedures before starting a woman on the Pill or inserting an IUD. Once the method is being used, the doctor will want to monitor progress. Medical supervision obviously includes physical examination and investigations.

Much ado has recently been made about taking a sexual history. A process akin to contact tracing has no place in the family planning consultation. Open-ended questions such as, 'Do you think you could be at risk of HIV infection?' are usually more revealing than closed questions such as 'How many sexual partners have you had?' If a doctor is very worried about the possibility of a sexually transmitted disease then the patient should clearly be referred to the genitourinary medicine clinic. Raising the subject of HIV in the consultation is relevant these days even if the patient does not feel so. A simple introduction is to mention that contraception can protect against pregnancy and infection. Methods such as barriers may do both jobs but patients and their partners will need to consider whether they need a highly effective contraceptive method combined with a barrier for protection against infection. With so much media coverage about HIV it is becoming easier to raise this subject but many patients will still feel they are not at risk.

SUMMARIZING

This is a short but important phase of the consultation which only Neighbour (1987) has separated out. The doctor summarizes in the patient's language what has been heard. This gives the patient an opportunity to check that the doctor has fully understood the problem and has taken into account her ideas, concerns, expectations and feelings. The patient has her own ideas about the nature of the problem, its causes, its importance and its possible outcomes. Likewise, the patient may have concerns, for instance that the Pill may cause some damage to her body. Or she may have expectations about the management of problems, such as that the doctor will refer her to a gynaecologist on account of breakthrough bleeding.

Summarizing provides direct feedback to the patient. If accepted, the consultation moves on. If not, the patient explains what it is that she feels the doctor has misinterpreted and then the doctor tries again.

NEGOTIATING A PLAN

Middleton's model consists of reconciling the patient's and doctor's agendas and drawing up a negotiated plan. The two agendas are not always compatible and it is well known that compliance is poor if the patient does not wholeheartedly back the plan of campaign. The days of giving out authoritarian, prescriptive advice are long since over. However, patients should be given up-to-date information on the different methods available and method teaching should be carried out.

Nearly one-half of all information given in general practice consultations is forgotten (Ley, 1982). Advice can be given in ways which increase the likelihood of the patient remembering it

(Fowler, 1985a). It is useful to stress important pieces of advice, using short words and sentences, giving specific rather than general advice and repeating advice. Countering myths is also important. The use of leaflets to supplement advice is vital (Fowler, 1985b). The Family Planning Information Service sets a very high standard with its set of family planning leaflets.

Included in this section is Neighbour's handing-over phase under which heading he includes negotiating with the patient, influencing the patient and how the plan is presented. Before moving on, it is necessary to check that the patient is happy with the plan. The patient should be encouraged to accept an appropriate degree of responsibility.

DISCUSSING FOLLOW-UP

Again, this phase is one from Neighbour's model (1987), although he calls it 'safety-netting', an expression which may not be immediately clear to everyone. This phase involves agreeing an outline of further management and the timing of the next appointment. Equally, it is important to make clear how to gain access to the doctor or nurse in the event of any difficulty, the symptoms which a patient should report immediately and the possibility of changing contraceptive method if the proposed method does not suit.

SELF-MONITORING

This process takes place continuously while a doctor is consulting but needs to be practised for full advantage to be gained. There are two elements. First, recognition of the feelings in the doctor engendered by the patient may help him or her to understand the patient's problems, particularly if a problem involves a relationship with another person. In Chapter 1, Elphis Christopher describes beautifully how the process of becoming entangled with the patient's problem allows feelings in the doctor to surface. Freeling and Harris (1984) categorize the doctor's feelings into those that are unconnected, indirectly connected and directly connected. Unconnected feelings can arise from the doctor's own domestic problems or from an emotion aroused by the last patient seen. Indirectly connected feelings may arise when the doctor identifies a problem he or she has experienced, such as a marital or sexual difficulty. Both of these categories of feeling lie strictly in the domain of the doctor's personal life. Directly connected feelings may be used legitimately in the consultation. Training in psychosexual medicine helps doctors to appreciate when it may be appropriate to feed these back to the patient. However, this must be done carefully and sensitively. This skill is an intuitive one which is a far cry from the conventional history-taking type of consultation that many doctors were taught at medical school.

The second purpose of self-monitoring is to avoid or allay stress in the doctor. Neighbour (1987) mentions various techniques either during or between consultations to reduce stress levels. For example, an exercise where one is aware of one's breathing can be used during a consultation and making a telephone call or reading the post are diversionary rituals which can be used between consultations. An aggressive patient may make us feel angry or upset and we owe it to the next patient to dissipate these feelings before we see them, as carry-over into the following consultation would be very unfair.

SATISFACTION

Little is known as yet about the outcome of consultations, but some work on satisfaction has been carried out (Ley, 1982). Only about two-thirds of patients in general practice are satisfied with communication within their consultations. Satisfied patients comply better with advice and have higher levels of recall of medical information. Qualities in the doctor which facilitate satisfaction are: being friendly rather than business-like; understanding the patient's concerns; and not thwarting the patient's expectations.

Numerous studies demonstrate deficiencies in communication skills among doctors (McAvoy, 1985). As high quality consultations appear to have far-reaching benefits, more effective teaching of such skills is needed.

CONCLUSION

Hopefully, this chapter has shown how radically doctors' consultations nowadays should differ from those of, say, 50 years ago. It seems that the fundamental elements are setting aside the illness/diagnosis model with its direct questions about bodily systems and adopting a patient-centred counselling style with its associated intuitive component. In this way doctors can not only elicit the real reasons why a patient is consulting them, but work out solutions together. By tackling problems at a deeper level doctors can learn from the relationships with their patients and help them to apply this understanding to other relationships. The doctor can then truly be said to be fulfilling his or her role as teacher, as the derivation of the word doctor implies.

REFERENCES

Balint, M. (1964) *The Doctor, His Patient and the Illness*, Pitman, London.

Byrne, P.S. and Long, B.E.L. (1976) *Doctors talking to Patients*, HMSO, London.

Fowler, C. (1985a) Health education in general practice: giving advice. *Health Education Journal*, **44**, 103–4.

Fowler, G. (1985b) Health education in general practice: the use of leaflets. *Health Education Journal*, **44**, 149–50

Freeling, P. and Harris, C.M. (1984) *The Doctor-Patient Relationship*, Churchill Livingstone, Edinburgh.

Heron, J. (1975) *Six Category Intervention Analysis*, University of Surrey, Guildford.

Ley, P. (1982) Satisfaction, compliance and communication. *British Journal of Clinical Psychology*, **21**, 241–54.

McAvoy, B.R. (1985) Communication skills and family planning doctors. *British Journal of Family Planning*, **11**, 44–9.

McEwan, J. (1982) Contraceptive advice in general practice. *Maternal and Child Health*, **7**, 470–4.

Middleton, J.E. (1989) The exceptional potential of the consultation revisited. *Journal of the Royal College of General Practitioners*, **39**, 383–6.

Neighbour, R. (1987) *The Inner Consultation*, MTP Press, Lancaster.

Pendleton, D., Schofield, T., Tate, P. *et al.* (1984) *The Consultation: An Approach to Learning and Teaching*, Oxford University Press, Oxford.

Pietroni, P. (1976) Nonverbal communication in the general practice surgery, in *Language and Communication in General Practice* (ed. B.A. Tanner), Hodder & Stoughton, London.

Stewart, M. and Woodhouse, J. (1987) What does the doctor wear? *British Journal of Family Planning*, **12**, 131–4.

Stott, N.C.H. and Davis, R.H. (1979) The exceptional potential in each primary care consultation. *Journal of the Royal College of General Practitioners*, **29**, 201-5.

Wilkinson, C. (1989) Time to let the patient speak. *British Medical Journal*, **298**, 389.

14

Seminar training for contraceptive care

Ruth Skrine

There is a road from the eye to the heart that does not go through the intellect.

G.K. Chesterton (1914)

We are thinking beings, and we cannot exclude the intellect from participating in any of our functions.

William James (reprinted 1982)

SUMMARY

- Doctor and patient's agenda revisited
- The seminar
- Unspoken communications
- Comfort with sexual matters
- What sort of doctor?
- The physical examination
- The body and the mind

The efficient and continuous use of contraception, and the choice of method, is not always an easy matter. The individual is affected by conscious ideas about the methods and about him or herself. Unconscious factors are of equal importance, and are complicated by the projective forces acting to varying degrees between the two members of every couple.

Contraception is about sexual feelings, and such feelings spring from, and are affected by, the deepest layers of the personality. As detailed earlier in this book, the provision of contraceptive care is not always as straightforward as it seems. However, what may appear at first as a heavy burden on the providing doctor or nurse can be viewed in a different light. The contraceptive consultation can provide an opportunity to reveal hidden anxieties and discomforts in the hope that some help will be forthcoming. Because contraception is inextricably connected to sex it can provide a communication pathway for the patient's deepest feelings. Using this pathway the patient may be able to reach outwards towards a professional person in the hope of finding help with an inner pain.

Sexual problems may be the underlying cause of individual ill health and unhappiness. The destructive effect of marital disharmony on children is well recognized. If anything can be done to lessen the stresses present in the family, the returns are likely to be great, although difficult to measure in a quantitative way. Certainly, any help that can be given to the parents of children should help to break the cycle of emotional deprivation, where those who have had insufficient nurture when young find it difficult to offer such nourishment to their children.

Most doctors and nurses have received little training about sexual matters during the course of their undergraduate years, and indeed it can be argued that such a training is better provided at the postgraduate stage when they are not so preoccupied with the exploration of their own sexuality. Chapter 13 gives an account of the different ways of studying the consultation process. One of the models outlined can be used to provide a framework within which the interaction between the patient and the doctor or nurse, can be examined at the time the events are taking place. The importance of developing doctors who can think about these happenings has been stressed by Norell, who says that the consultation should be considered as an organic entity (Norell, 1984). Marinker suggests that not all consultations are problem solving, but that some are more like 'a piece of theatre, a celebration or an expiation'; not to be valued as crosswords but more as poems (Marinker, 1986). The intuitive side of the consultation, suggested in the quotation from Chesterton above, has been explored by Neighbour, as mentioned in Chapter 13.

Such an approach can become vague and sentimental if it is not balanced by a rigorous use of the intellect.

DOCTOR AND PATIENT'S AGENDA REVISITED

Thinking about the consultation makes the doctor aware of the differences between his or her agenda and that of the patient. Opportunities can then be made for the patient to express her or his own ideas and anxieties. The patient's agenda may consist of fairly straightforward questions that are easily asked provided the doctor allows enough silence and space. Some anxieties are too personal or embarrassing to be broached directly, and the variety of calling cards and presenting symptoms is well known. Such calling cards are particularly common where the underlying anxiety is to do with sexual matters, and contraceptive problems are one of the commonest presentations. However, many underlying difficulties are even less conscious, and may only be guessed at by recognizing inappropriate or inconsistent behaviour. The doctor's agenda might include a wish to understand some of this behaviour, for instance, what makes it impossible for a couple to find any effective method of contraception, or why a young girl is asking for her third termination. What skills does the doctor need in order to be able to explore such matters, and how may these skills be obtained?

THE SEMINAR

Balint (1957) was the pioneer of the study of interactions between doctors and patients, and his group training methods have been used widely. Originally, the groups were led by psychoanalysts who were not themselves general practitioners, and whose concern was not the teaching of general practice, but the running of a group where problems met by general practitioners could be studied. Within the Institute of Psychosexual Medicine, Main has extended Balint's ideas by training doctors experienced in psychosexual medicine, who are not themselves psychoanalysts, to be the leaders of groups where the question of psychosomatic sexuality can be studied.

The method of training is based on case discussion of the member's ongoing clinical work, and is aimed at developing skills rather than instilling knowledge (Main, 1983). Group members may be disappointed at the length of time it takes to acquire new attitudes and skills. It is important to stress that these groups are not for supervision, where members come for advice about what to do with their patients, but opportunities to think afresh about what is going on in the consultation. The responsibility for the management of the patient remains with the doctor at all times.

If doctors are to offer help they must be able to listen to, and empathize with, the feelings of their patients. Most doctors have built up some form of protective emotional shell to defend themselves from the pain and suffering that they have had to witness during their time as students and hospital doctors. Some such shell is necessary for their personal survival, but if there is no opportunity for them to allow themselves to recognize their feelings, they will be poor whole-person doctors.

The use of a consultation model can be a way of encouraging doctors to think about what is going on in the consultation. Seminar training extends that process. The act of telling the story of the patient and the troubles, in as far as they can be remembered, and expressing his or her own reactions to that story, helps the doctor to 'acquire a measure of psychological distance from the engagement of himself and his patient together in treatment' (Gosling, Miller, Woodhouse *et al.*, 1967). Such engagement, referred to as the doctor/patient relationship, is the focus for the work of the group. The seminar experience encourages the doctor to let himself or herself feel, then pull back and think about those feelings. If the feelings are truly experienced, thinking stops momentarily; conversely, it is difficult to feel deeply when thinking. The process is one of constant change between these two positions as the act of pulling back to think can allow more feeling to follow, and as more is felt there is more to think about.

UNSPOKEN COMMUNICATIONS

The process of thinking during a consultation, and subsequently describing what happened to a group of colleagues, soon leads to an awareness of many unspoken communications from the patient. Mode of dress, the presence or absence of eye contact, feelings of anger, despair or withdrawal coming from the patient are reported by the doctor. But, more importantly, the doctor begins to be able to study the feelings that are present in himself or herself, and to see that they may have been aroused by the particular patient in the consulting room. Thus it is the interaction, the atmosphere, the flow of feeling and action between the two people that is the subject of study and that can reveal unconscious truths about the patient. One doctor in training said, 'I am learning to use another part of myself to help my patients.'

A flow of feeling cannot occur if the doctor spends the whole time asking questions or giving advice, and he or she learns to allow the patient to choose the subject matter by a judicious use of open-ended questions and encouraging signs. As has been mentioned in Chapter 13, such an approach can take less time and is more appropriate to a primary care consultation than a traditional medical history. A simple example of the efficient use of time is to ask the patient how she feels about starting on the Pill. One trainee doctor spent ten minutes explaining in great detail all the thrombotic and cancer risks and benefits of the Pill while the patient's eyes glassed over. When asked at the end what *her* anxieties were, she said she was worried about her future fertility. The doctor's time could have been spent more profitably dealing with the patient's anxieties rather than going through a required formula to which she was not listening.

During a short family planning consultation in general practice or in a clinic it will, of course, be necessary to ask some questions and to give some advice, but the timing of such activity is worth studying. Is it an appropriate moment to move on with the practicalities, or has the doctor escaped into 'traditional doctoring' because of some discomfort between doctor and patient? Noticing, thinking about and possibly commenting on that discomfort rather than running away from it can provide a further space for the patient to reveal hidden feelings.

COMFORT WITH SEXUAL MATTERS

For many doctors, as for their patients, sex is a private, personal and sometimes embarrassing topic. Most people have sexual anxieties or disappointments at some time in their lives, but the majority are able to overcome them or adapt to them with, if they are lucky, the help of a loving partner. However, whether we like it or not, when working in the contraceptive field all doctors and nurses will meet patients who ask for help with their sexual lives either overtly or covertly. The doctor's personal experience gives him or her a sensitivity to the patient's feelings, and possible insight into the general difficulties of patients. However, they are of no help in understanding the particular patient in that consultation as each person and each problem is unique. It must be stressed that at no time are doctors in seminar training expected or encouraged to talk about their own sexuality. The group is not there to provide therapy for the doctor, and any personal help that is gained, or change that may take place, is a private matter for that doctor.

However, discussion of sexual matters in the seminar can make the subject more comfortable. Doctors attending seminars have said that it is a safe place in which to practice the discussion of sexual details, and they gain greater confidence to listen to, or to broach sexual topics with their patients.

Setting clear training boundaries that exclude personal sexual revelations and that tie all discussion to a specific case, allows for a study of those difficult moments in the consultation when a feeling of sexiness develops in the room. For the woman doctor faced with a man who produces an erection, the embarrassment can be great for both parties. It may be possible to see such moments as unconsicous defences on the part of the patient (Skrine, 1987). Certainly the doctor is usually de-skilled and has to retreat to the safety of the prescription pad, the ordering of tests or a referral to another doctor. During training the doctor can learn to cope with such moments with some degree of equanimity.

A male doctor was faced with a patient whose calling card was a rather vague account of irregular bleeding on the Pill. The doctor noticed that she seemed rather withdrawn and unhappy. In response to a general enquiry about other worries she began to tell him about the sexual abuse she had suffered from her father in her early teens. Suddenly the doctor noticed that she appeared overwhelmingly attractive. The strength of his feelings in response made him stop listening to what she was saying. He reported to the group that he was able to recognize his own feelings, and the fact that they had stopped him listening. He managed to say nothing to the patient, and resolved to make himself listen to her story some more. Gradually, the sense of sexiness wore off, and by the end of the consultation he felt comfortable enough to consider the possibility of a genital examination without anxiety.

During discussion the group noticed how the flirtatiousness of the patient had appeared suddenly at the time that she was talking about her abuse. With the knowledge that abused people often find the maintenance of boundaries difficult, it was possible to understand that she might have difficulties maintaining the boundaries of a professional relationship with her doctor. Thanks to his training the doctor was able to stay with the difficult moment, not run away or attack, and provide an experience for the patient of a man in authority who could tolerate her flirtatiousness without responding to it.

WHAT SORT OF DOCTOR?

If the reactions between the patient and the doctor are to be studied as a way of illuminating the patient's problem, it is necessary for the doctor to be aware of his or her normal doctoring style. It is then possible to recognize changes from this norm, and to think about what it is in the patient that has provoked that change. Such a way of thinking is very different from the way the doctor has previously been trained where the emphasis was on the collection of accurate information, logical thinking about differential diagnosis and the provision of correct treatment.

Doctors come into seminars hoping to learn how to help people with contraceptive or psychosomatic difficulties. Their thinking is concerned with, 'Was my action right or wrong?' or 'How could I have done better?' Gradually they learn to think differently, and to wonder, 'What was it about the patient that made me act in that way?' Or to put it another way, 'What sort of doctor was I to that patient?' Such questions can lead to a re-examination of the patient's problem, often providing clues to unconscious forces that had not previously been recognized. For instance, a doctor may become much more of a didactic teacher than usual.

A young mother came to a family planning clinic asking to go back on the Pill. She admitted that before the pregnancy she had often forgotten to take the Pills for two or three days at a time. The doctor, who normally listens well, found herself giving a lecture about the importance of regular Pill taking, especially now she had a young baby to care for. When the doctor and nurse discussed the patient later it was discovered that the nurse, too, had lectured the patient in a more didactic way than was normal for her.

Something in this patient had provoked her two carers to treat her as a child, telling her what to do rather than exploring her feelings and the reasons behind her actions. No attempt had been made to discover why she used to miss Pills, or whether the situation was likely to be the same now. If there was a degree of immaturity in the patient that made it difficult for her to appreciate the possible outcome of her actions, that missing Pills could lead to pregnancy, how helpful was it to continue to treat her as a child? Is that the way to encourage maturity and self-care? If she was missing Pills because of an unconscious need to get pregnant, a recognition of that need might have helped her to better use contraception in the future.

Sometimes doctors are given second chances, and it is possible that the belated recognition of the 'teacher' who was provoked in the doctor and nurse by the patient will make it possible to explore the 'childish' behaviour at the next visit.

Other feelings in the doctor can be seen to have developed in response to the patient. Irritability, anger and even a particular degree of sadness or despair become subjects of study. Indeed, the feelings may be projected from the patient, via the presenting doctor, into the group. For instance, unconscious aspects of the patient may be seen particularly clearly when her or his ambivalent feelings reveal themselves by a split in the feelings and sympathies of the group members themselves.

An anxiety for many doctors and nurses is the fear that they may have to discuss their own personal feelings in the group. It has already been pointed out that at no time is the sexuality of the professional a subject of study. Similarly, the members are not required to look at their own history or hang-ups in the group, but only at their doctoring or nursing skills. There is no sense in which doctors have to 'fully understand themselves' before they can help patients, for if that were so there would be few doctors working in this way. Most of those whose personal difficulties are so severe as to interfere with their work will not join a group, or they will soon opt out.

Members learn to make allowances for their own private biases within the privacy of their own personal lives. A few who find that the group experience stirs up personal difficulties will seek personal help outside the group.

THE PHYSICAL EXAMINATION

Doctors, nurses and some other health professionals such as physiotherapists are in the unique position of having licence to examine the most intimate parts of the body; indeed, they are expected and required to do so. The vulnerable moment of examination may provide an opportunity for the patient to get in touch with feelings. Sometimes she has been aware of the feelings but has not been able to share them before. Sometimes she may be surprised by feelings she did not even know that she had. In this context the word 'she' is appropriate, as the finding was first noticed with women and thought to be particularly potent because of the hidden nature of the female genitalia (Tunnadine, 1992). One woman, at the moment that the labia were parted by the doctor, said, 'There is an inner and outer part of me . . . the curtains have to be parted . . . I cannot find my female self.' Revelations can also take place during the examination of other parts of the body, especially the breasts. However, the finding is not confined to women; important moments of emotional contact are also experienced during the examination of the man, and particularly his genitals (Barrett, 1992).

Noticing the emotional content, or the lack of it, at the time of a physical genital examination is a psychosomatic skill. When the details of the examination are studied they always provide some information about the patient, even if it is only to do with the degree of control of detachment. But it is not a prying examination on the part of the doctor to discover secrets that the patient wishes to hide. Rather it is an enabling moment when the patient may be able to get in touch with unacknowledged feelings. Often it is the moment when some unspoken anxiety can be revealed, and there is an opportunity for the doctor and patient together to explore her ideas and fantasies about the body.

During a routine Pill check consultation the patient mentioned that she had experienced painful intercourse since the birth of her baby six years previously. She believed that she had been 'ripped', and that the stitches had come undone. She had already consulted two gynaecologists who were loathe to undertake any surgery as she appeared well healed. As the doctor looked at the healed but scarred perineum, noticing the scar tissue was a lighter and pinker colour than the slightly pigmented skin on either side of it, the patient said that she had looked at it in the mirror and there was no 'space' between the front and back passages. What she seemed to be saying was that the vagina and rectum felt to her to be joined, with no wall between them. It is interesting that she had also been complaining of a lot of wind which she felt was 'getting in from below'. There was a sense that air was getting from the rectum to the vagina and thence 'to the insides'.

Once the patient had been helped to put these ideas into words, it was not difficult to help her to confront her fantasy with the reality of a intact vagina by encouraging her to feel inside and to contract her muscles round her finger.

In the seminar doctors learn how important it is to identify and pay tribute to the specific body fantasy. One young woman, unable to make love since the birth of her last baby three years before, had already had two reconstructive operations to her perineum. She described her sense that each time she was stitched up the hole got smaller, 'like cobbling up a hole in a stocking. If I had six children there would be no hole left'.

The moment of physical examination can be a time when deep feelings are shared. Such feelings include anger and grief, and it is surprising how much bereavement work goes on in the family planning consultation. The losses of miscarriage and termination might be expected, but it is not unusual for a patient to share such anguishes as the death of a parent. The moment of physical examination may trigger renewed grieving, as has been described previously (Montford, 1992).

THE BODY AND THE MIND

General practitioners are familiar with the idea that illnesses are seldom due to purely physical or purely emotional causes. The input of each side has to be weighed at every consultation. Seminar training can foster the skill of keeping an open mind, and promote the study of the interaction between the body and the mind, which is especially important in the sexual area of the patient's life.

Psychosexual skills are not a watered down form of psychotherapy, although psychodynamic ideas are used in the training and practice. The doctor develops a focused way of working in an important area of the patient's emotional life. Those in training will probably want to arrange times when they can give their patients a few longer appointments, but they are not encouraged to engage in extended therapy. Indeed, the doctor/patient relationship where the doctor becomes over-involved with the patient is worthy of study, and may be revealing a particular problem of dependency for that patient. The aim of training is not to suggest that doctors should provide time-consuming long-term support, which may be more appropriately provided by others, but that they should learn to use specific skills within the practice of their normal work. The general practice and clinic settings, and particularly the family planning consultation, provide patients with repeated opportunities to visit doctors about routine matters, and they can choose the moment that is appropriate for them to discuss their inner pains.

Doctors learn to look for and think about direct clinical evidence in the 'here and now' of the consultation. Such evidence can provide powerful hints about the patient's predicament. If and when the patient chooses to talk about past relationships and memories, these will have been remembered because they have special meaning for the patient in the present. They are then far more relevant to the current problem than answers provided in reply to questions about the past history.

The most important skill that doctors learn in seminars is to tolerate not knowing. Neither the patient nor the docor has the truth, which has been described as 'a reality that exists in between; in between two people seeking it; in between psychoanalysis, sociology, psychology, economics and religion ... truth can be seen or glimpsed, not possessed' (Symington, 1986). Psychosexual doctors learn to stay in ignorance with their patients, searching for a glimpse of the truth, for as T.S. Elliott (1954) says in his poem *East Coker*

In order to arrive at what you know
You must go by a way which is a way of ignorance.
In order to possess what you do not possess
You must go by the way of dispossession.

Psychosexual medicine as it is understood in great Britain in the 1990s has come a long way from its roots in family planning, when the patient was usually a woman attending on her own. Help is now offered to men and to couples. Seminar training and research has furthered doctors' understanding of body–mind doctoring, and given insight into the skills that are needed to help patients in trouble with their sexual lives. It is worth remembering that the first psycho-sexual seminars were started in response to requests from doctors working in contraception who felt inadequate when they were faced with the sexual and emotional problems of their patients. Such problems are no less common today, and the sense of inadequacy is always present. As Main (1983) has said, '... every generation of doctors will demand a training, because doctors are never satisfied with their skills. In their discontent lies hope for the next generation of patients.'

REFERENCES

Balint, M. (1957) *The Doctor, His Patient and the Illness*, Pitman Medical Publishing, London.

Barrett, P. (1992) Impotence: the referred patient, in *Psychosexual Medicine* (ed. Lincoln), Chapman & Hall, London.

Chesterton, G.K. (1914) *The Defendant*, J.M. Dent, London.

Eliot, T.S. (1954) *Four Quartets*, Faber & Faber, London.

Gosling, R., Miller, D.H., Woodhouse, D. *et al.* (1967) *The Use of Small Groups in Training*, Codicote Press, London.

James, W. (reprinted 1982) *The Varieties of Religious Experience*, Harmondsworth, London.

Main, T. (1983) Training for acquisition of knowledge or development of skill? in *The Practice of Psychosexual Medicine* (ed. K. Draper), John Libbey, London.

Marinker, M. (1986) Workshop in research and communication, Institute of Psychosexual Medicine. *Newsletter*, 7–11 November (limited circulation available from the Institute).

232   *Seminar training for contraceptive care*

Montford, H. (1992) Pelvic pain and dyspareunia, in *Psychosexual Medicine* (ed. Lincoln), Chapman & Hall, London.

Norell, J. (1984) What every doctor knows. *Journal of the Royal College of General Practitioners*, **34**, 417–24.

Skrine, R. (ed.) (1987) Sexualizing the interview, in *Psychosexual Training and the Doctor/Patient Relationship*, Chapman & Hall, London.

Symington, N. (1986) *The Analytic Experience*, Free Association Books, London.

Tunnadine, P. (1992) *Insights into Troubled Sexuality*, Chapman & Hall, London.

Index

Index

Index